Handbook of Pain Management

Editor
Michael Serpell
Consultant and Senior Lecturer in Anaesthesia,
University Department of Anaesthesia,
Gartnavel General Hospital, Glasgow, Scotland

Contributors
Mike Basler
Consultant in Anaesthesia and Pain Medicine,
Department of Anaesthesia,
Glasgow Royal Infirmary, Glasgow, Scotland

Maheshwar Chaudhari
Consultant in Anaesthesia and Pain Management,
Sheffield Teaching Hospitals NHS Trust,
Sheffield, UK

Martin Dunbar
Clinical Psychologist,
Department of Anaesthetics,
Stobhill Hospital, Glasgow, Scotland

Jonathan McGhie
Consultant in Anaesthesia and Pain Management,
University Department of Anaesthesia,
Gartnavel General Hospital, Glasgow, Scotland

Lars Williams
Consultant in Anaesthesia and Pain Management,
Department of Anaesthesia,
Southern General Hospital, Glasgow, Scotland

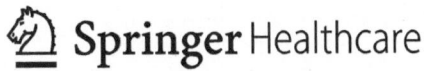

Published by Springer Healthcare Ltd, 236 Gray's Inn Road, London, WC1X 8HB, UK

www.springerhealthcare.com

British Library Cataloguing-in-Publication Data.
A catalogue record for this book is available from the British Library.
ISBN 978-1-85873-410-1

Although every effort has been made to ensure that drug doses and other information are presented accurately in this publication, the ultimate responsibility rests with the prescribing physician. Neither the publisher nor the authors can be held responsible for errors or for any consequences arising from the use of the information contained herein. Any product mentioned in this publication should be used in accordance with the prescribing information prepared by the manufacturers. No claims or endorsements are made for any drug or compound at present under clinical investigation.

Commissioning editor: Dinah Alam
Project editor: Alison Whitehouse
Designer: Joe Harvey
Production: Marina Maher

Contents

Author biographies

Mike Basler, MBChB, FRCA, FFPMANZCA is a consultant in Anaesthetics and Pain Management in Glasgow, Scotland. He trained in anaesthetics in the UK and, following completion of pain training in Adelaide, Australia, became a fellow of the Faculty of Pain Medicine. He took up his consultant post in 1999.

He is currently the Honorary Secretary of the North British Pain Association and writes an editorial column for the newsletter of the British Pain Society. He is the Pain Management representative on the Association of Anaesthetists Scottish Board and has worked with NHS Quality Improvement Scotland on several documents pertaining to chronic pain management. He is the Acute Pain Editor of the Anaesthesia section of the National Electronic Library for Health. His interests include burn pain, neuropathic pain and invasive cancer pain management.

Maheshwar Chaudhari, MD, FRCA, DPM is a consultant in Anaesthesia and Pain Management at Sheffield Teaching Hospitals NHS Trust, Sheffield, UK. He graduated from B. J. Medical College, Pune, India. He completed his postgraduate training in Anaesthesia (MD) at Jiwaji University, Gwalior, India, and then worked as a registrar in Anaesthetics at Safdarjung Hospital, New Delhi. He underwent SHO training in Anaesthesia at Peterborough Hospitals NHS Trust, Peterborough, UK, before becoming a senior specialist registrar in Anaesthesia and Pain Management in the West Midlands region.

After completing his Fellowship examination, he did advanced pain training at Glasgow and achieved a Diploma in Pain Medicine. His main interests in anaesthesia are regional anaesthesia and chronic pain management.

Martin Dunbar, BSc(Hons), PhD, DClinPsychol is a clinical psychologist. He took his first degree in psychology in London, graduating in 1989. Following this he moved to Edinburgh to do his PhD. From 1992 to 1998 he worked as a non-clinical scientist at the MRC Social and Public Health Sciences Unit at Glasgow University, Scotland. He then underwent clinical psychology training in Edinburgh, qualifying in 2001. Since then he has been working in the pain service in Glasgow.

He currently provides clinical psychology support to two pain clinics at hospitals in the north of Glasgow as well as working in the Glasgow Back Pain Service where his clinical focus is on the prevention of chronic pain. He is the clinical psychology representative on the council of the North British

Pain Association and has joint responsibility for organizing their scientific meetings. His research interests are in the broad area of the interface between psychology and medicine.

Jonathan McGhie, MB ChB, FRCA, FFPMANZCA graduated in medicine from the University of Glasgow, Scotland, in 1998. He trained in Anaesthetics in Glasgow, and completed his pain training in Sydney, Australia, where he became a fellow of the Australian Faculty of Pain Medicine by examination.

He took up a consultant post in Glasgow in 2007 and is interested in chronic pain, cancer pain and pain training. He has previously contributed to book chapters on the pharmacology of local anaesthetics and on postoperative neuropathic pain. He participates in the Glasgow pain education group that develops pain training in the west of Scotland and has been involved in establishing a tutorial programme for the pain trainees.

Michael Serpell, MB ChB, FCPodS, ECFMG, FRCA graduated from Medical School at the University of Dundee in 1983. He completed his training in Anaesthesia and Pain Management in Dundee, Scotland, Orebro in Sweden and Dartmouth Hitchcock Medical Centre in New Hampshire, USA. He took up his consultant post in Glasgow in 1993 and became Senior Lecturer at the University Department of Anaesthesia, Glasgow in 1999.

His research interests include pharmacological and regional analgesia management of acute and chronic pain. He is particularly interested in the diagnosis and early treatment of neuropathic pain. He leads the Clinical Trials Unit at the Pain Clinic in Gartnavel, which runs both acute and chronic pain studies. He is Chairman of the Research and Priority Programme for Pain and Acute Medicine for the Greater Glasgow Acute Hospitals Trust. He is Chairman of the Local Arrangements Committee for the IASP World Congress on Pain to be held in Glasgow, August 2008. He is Chairman of the Neuropathic Pain Specialist Interest Group of the British Pain Society, and Examiner for the Primary FRCA. He has been Secretary and Treasurer of the North British Pain Association and Secretary of the West of Scotland Pain Group.

He is Senior Series Editor of *Anaesthesia and Intensive Care Medicine* and is its Speciality Editor in Pain. He is an Associate Editor for the *European Journal of Pain* and a reviewer for several journals, including *British Journal of Anaesthesia*. He is Block Editor for Pain for the Royal College of Anaesthetists' electronic Learning in Anaesthesia (eLA) project. He has published 15 chapters and over 40 original research papers. He was a member of a team that received an Art-Science grant from the Wellcome Foundation to co-produce a play about chronic pain – *PUSH* – which was performed in London during June 2003.

Lars Williams, MB, ChB, FRCA, studied medicine at Aberdeen University, UK, qualifying MB, ChB in 1991. After a spell working in psychiatry he began training in anaesthesia, first in Birmingham, UK, then Glasgow, Scotland. His training included a year in Melbourne, Australia, and a year as a clinical fellow in pain medicine, West of Scotland School of Anaesthesia. He took up his post as Consultant in Anaesthesia and Pain Management in Glasgow in 2004.

Dr Williams chairs the West of Scotland Pain Group and is responsible for coordinating training in pain management for the West of Scotland School of Anaesthesia. He has a major clinical interest in pain management, including clinical input to the Glasgow pain management programme and involvement in a developing intrathecal therapy service for cancer pain. He has recently completed the Diploma in Pain Management at the University of Wales College of Medicine, UK. Research interests include the use of diagnostic drug infusion tests, trainee assessment and clinical informatics in pain management.

Chapter 1

Introduction

Pain and quality of life

Pain is a complex interaction that involves sensory, emotional and behavioural factors, and so its definition and treatment must include all of these aspects. The International Association for the Study of Pain's (IASP's) definition of pain is 'an unpleasant sensory and emotional experience associated with potential or actual tissue damage' [1].

Pain has numerous detrimental effects. Acute pain is a core component of the stress response to injury, and therefore should be managed aggressively and appropriately in order to reduce these effects and optimize patient recovery and minimize complications (*see* Figure 1.1).

Pain not only results in mental suffering, but also has a negative impact on the general activity and function of the patient. The amount of dysfunction is not linearly related to the amount of pain. Two people can have identical pain scores from identical causes, for example after hernia surgery, and

Figure 1.1 Pathophysiological associations of pain	
CNS	Inhumane, misery, anxiety, depression, sleep disturbance
CVS	↑ Blood pressure, heart rate and vascular resistance, ↑ cardiac ischaemia
RESP	Cough inhibition (pneumonia), hyperventilation (respiratory alkalosis)
GIT	Ileus, nausea, vomiting
GUS	Urinary retention, uterine inhibition
Muscle	Restless – ↑ oxygen consumption Immobility – ↑ incidence of pulmonary thromboembolism
Metabolic	– ↑ Catabolic: cortisone, glucagon, growth hormone, catecholamines – ↓ Anabolic: insulin, testosterone – ↑ Plasminogen activator inhibitor (↑ coagulation)

CNS, central nervous system; CVS, cardiovascular system; GIT, gastrointestinal tract; GUS, genitourinary system; RESP, respiratory system.

Figure 1.2 Relationship between functional impairment[a] and pain score[b]

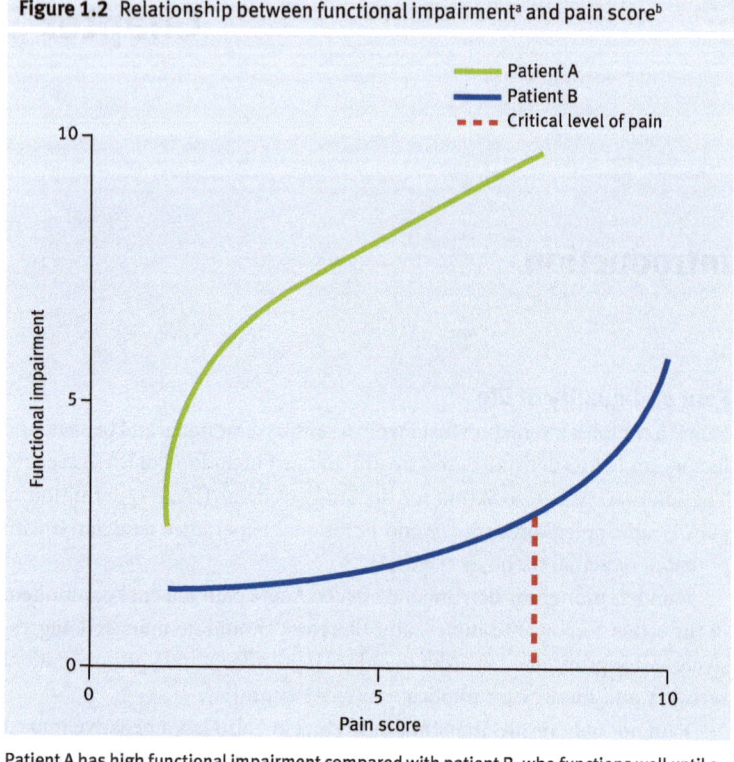

Patient A has high functional impairment compared with patient B, who functions well until a critical level of pain is reached.
[a]0 = none, 10 = severe; [b]0 = none, 10 = worst.

yet have totally different levels of impairment (*see* Figure 1.2). The reason for this is that we are all individuals and we respond differently to the challenge of pain.

Chronic pain has an even greater detrimental effect on function and quality of life as the relentless suffering can result in severe anxiety, depression and behavioural changes. This can result in the patient suffering irreversible loss of identity and function within their domestic, social and professional roles (*see* Figure 1.3).

Definitions of pain [2]

Acute versus chronic pain. There is an arbitrary cut-off point of 3 months that distinguishes the two [1]. However, the consensus is that pain is defined as chronic if it persists for longer than is reasonably expected. For example, pain

Figure 1.3 Cancer pain: increasing pain scores reflect more severe and non-linear functional interference*

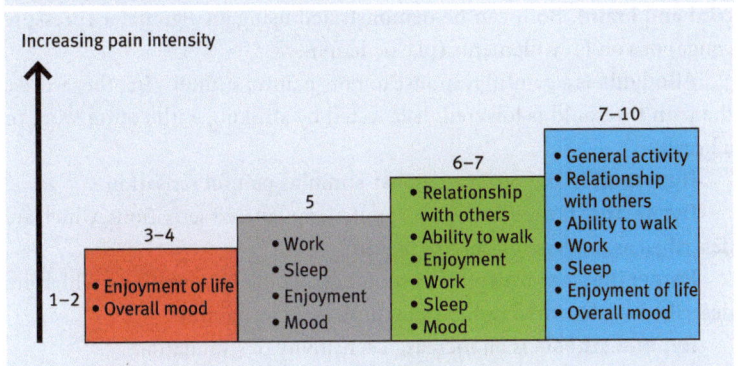

*P<0.001.
Data from Breitbart W, Bruera E, Chochinov H, Lynch M. Neuropsychiatric syndromes and psychological symptoms in patients with advanced cancer. J Pain Symptom Manage 1995; 10:131–41.

from a simple tissue laceration should recede within a few weeks, whereas that from major and multiple trauma would be expected to take many months to settle. In the former case, if pain persists for more than even 6 weeks, an aggressive approach should be adopted to identify and manage any factors likely to maintain chronicity. This does not mean that severe pain caused by something like multiple trauma should be ignored for many months; it should also be aggressively managed. But often with severe trauma there may be ongoing causes of pain which will persist and maintain the nociceptive process until the tissue has predominantly healed. The aim here should be to expedite the healing while providing optimal analgesia.

Pain threshold is the minimal stimulus required to produce a cortical response on 50% of occasions. It follows a normal distribution and is reproducible, for example heat pain is most commonly perceived at 44°C. It is a useful scientific tool.

Pain tolerance is the maximum noxious stimulation that a patient will tolerate, i.e. it is the pain that patients actually complain about. It is less reproducible than pain threshold measurements. Pain tolerance is measured by a sub-maximal effort tourniquet test or pain visual analogue scale (VAS).

Hyperalgesia is an increased painful response to a stimulus that is normally painful – in other words, the response is amplified. Primary hyperalgesia results from stimulation of sensitized polymodal nociceptors within 5–10 mm of the area of injury. Secondary hyperalgesia is demonstrated outwith the area of peripheral nerve innervation (10–20 cm beyond) and results from mechanisms within the central nervous system (CNS) (spinal cord and brain). Both can be demonstrated using an algometer (pressure gauge) or von Frey filaments (plastic hairs).

Allodynia is a painful response to non-painful stimuli – in other words, the pain threshold is lowered. It is tested by stroking with cotton wool or a brush.

Hyperpathia is a prolonged post-stimulus painful sensation.

Dysaesthesiae are evoked or spontaneous altered sensations, which are described as unpleasant but not painful.

Paraesthesiae are evoked or spontaneous altered sensations, which are described as abnormal rather than unpleasant or painful.

Hyperaesthesia is an increased sensitivity of stimulation.

Clinical classification

Rather than separating types of pain into separate forms, the different types are now considered to be spread out along a spectrum. At one end is pure neuropathic pain, for example post-herpetic neuralgia (PHN) and painful diabetic neuropathy (PDN). At the other is pure nociceptive pain such as osteo- and rheumatoid arthritis. In between are a large number of pains that have a mixture (combination pain) of the two types, to varying degrees of predominance (*see* Figure 1.4).

Nociceptive pain

Somatic pain. This originates from skin, muscle and bone tissues. Physiological pain is a protective event that enables the organism rapidly and accurately to localize pain and withdraw from the stimulus in order to avoid or reduce further tissue damage. It is conveyed by myelinated Aδ-fibres, which then relay via the neospinothalamic tract to the somatosensory post-central gyrus at the cortex. If the stimulus is of short duration and does not cause tissue damage, the pain disappears when the stimulus stops.

Figure 1.4 The spectrum of combination pain

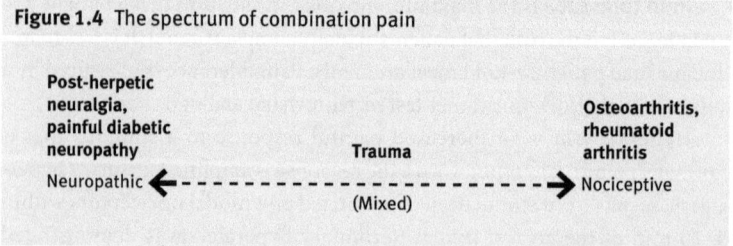

Pathophysiological pain is responsible for the delayed pain sensation that occurs after tissue injury (surgery, trauma and inflammation) and that encourages tissue healing by eliciting behaviour to protect the damaged area. This is the type of pain that health carers endeavour to manage. It is transmitted via unmyelinated C-fibres which then synapse and ascend cranially via the paleospinothalamic tract. It has collaterals that project to various structures in the brain (see Chapter 3). This system is primarily involved with reflex responses concerned with respiration, circulation and endocrine function. They also engage descending modulatory systems and all are involved in producing the emotional and behavioural response to pain.

Visceral pain. The density of visceral nociceptors is less than 1% in comparison with somatic afferents, and the cortical mapping of visceral afferents is also less concentrated. Therefore visceral pain is poorly localized, diffuse and frequently in the midline, with the exception of joints and the mesentery. The pain is commonly described as dull cramping, squeezing or dragging, which often occurs periodically, building up to peaks. There are often associated phenomena such as nausea or vomiting, perspiration, blood pressure and heart rate changes because of sympathetic innervations.

The qualitative nature of the pain is very different, in that the viscera are very sensitive to distension. It also appears that afferent fibres respond in a graded fashion to intensity of stimulation rather than to individual stimulating modalities. Furthermore, visceral pain exhibits spatial summation in that, if a large area is stimulated, the pain threshold is lowered, which does not occur in cutaneous somatic nociception.

Visceral pain can also be referred to a site far away from the source of stimulation. Referred pain is often segmental and superficial, and frequently shows hyperalgesia, for example bladder pain can produce these effects in the perianal S2–4 dermatomes.

Neuropathic pain

Injury to nerve fibres can lead to abnormal functioning of the nervous system. Complete destruction, for example following nerve transection, usually results in complete loss of sensation and motor function. Partial damage from physical injury (e.g. crush injury or following surgery) or medical conditions (e.g. diabetes or shingles) can result in the preservation of gross motor and sensory function but produce subtle abnormalities such as altered temperature sensation, unusual or unpleasant feelings, or even pain (see Figure 1.5). This altered function occurs because the overall activity of the nervous system results from the balance between excitatory and

Figure 1.5 Characteristics of neuropathic damage*

Negative phenomena	Positive phenomena
Sensory	
Hypoaesthesia	Hyperaesthesia, dysaesthesia
	Paraesthesia
Hypoalgesia	Hyperalgesia, hyperpathia, allodynia
Autonomic	
Vasodilatation	Vasoconstriction
Hypohidrosis, anhidrosis	Hyperhidrosis, piloerection
Motor	
Paralysis, paresis	Fasciculations, dystonia

*Only detectable for cutaneous nerves.

inhibitory components. Partial damage often leads to an increased activity and excitation of the nerve fibres. Therefore the thrust of treatment is suppression of this hyperactivity (*see* Chapter 4).

Psychogenic pain

Psychogenic pain is actually very uncommon, so those patients who are told that their pain 'is all in their head' are being unjustly managed. It is true that some psychiatric disorders can present with pain as the predominant complaint. For example, 30% of patients with clinical depression also complain of pain, which disappears once the depression has been successfully treated. However the other symptoms of depression are usually obvious and the diagnosis is often very clear. In somatoform disorders, the diagnosis is more difficult to make and requires specialist psychiatric examination utilizing DSM-IV (*Diagnostic and Statistical Manual of Mental Disorders*, 4th edition) [3] criteria.

Much more common is the association of pain and psychological pathology. It is inappropriate to see pain as either physical or psychological. It is always both, as stated in the IASP definition of pain [1]. The pain experienced and amount of suffering is dependent on many psychological parameters such as anxiety, past experiences, the meaning to the patient of the pain, injury or illness, their beliefs about treatment and medications (fear of dependence, addiction, tolerance, organ damage, etc.), and self-management strategies. This applies equally to acute and chronic pain, and so pain services should screen patients to address any critical psychological issues as an integral component of appropriate medical management. Motivation and positive attitudes can be just as important to pain control and recovery.

'Idiopathic' pain

'Idiopathic pain' means that the cause of pain is not obvious; it accounts for about one-fifth of patients in most chronic pain clinics. There may well be a list of suspected causes, but nothing to explain the severity of the pain or resulting dysfunction. A common example is chronic low back pain, which can occur with minimal structural or degenerative changes in the vertebral column. However, just because blood test profiles or imaging investigations are negative does not mean that there is no cause for pain. It is now well established that there are multiple abnormalities occurring at the cellular level that will not be detected by conventional investigations (*see* Chapter 3). Therefore pain 'is what the patient says it is', and it must be treated as a genuine symptom until proven otherwise.

References

1. Merskey H, Bogduk N (eds). Classification of Chronic Pain: Descriptions of Chronic Pain Syndromes and Definitions of Pain Terms, 2nd edn. IASP Task Force on Taxonomy. Seattle, WA: IASP Press, 1994, 209–14.
2. Bonica JJ (ed.). Definitions and Taxonomy of Pain. The Management of Pain, Vol. 1. Philadelphia, PA: Lea & Febiger, 1990, 20–1.
3. American Psychiatric Association. Diagnostic and Statistical Manual of Mental Disorders, 4th edn. Washington DC: American Psychiatric Association, 1994.

Further reading

Holdcroft A, Jaggar S (eds). Core Topics in Pain. Cambridge: Cambridge University Press, 2005.
Rowbotham DJ, Macintyre PE (eds). Clinical Pain Management – Acute Pain. London: Arnold, 2003.

Chapter 2

Anatomy and physiology of pain

Introduction

The unpleasant sensation of pain plays an important protective role. Physiological, 'fast' pain warns us of imminent tissue damage and enables us to locate and withdraw from the source of injury. Later, inflammatory, 'slow' pain encourages protective immobilization of the injured area, which promotes tissue healing and functional recovery.

Distinct from the subjective experience of pain, *nociception* describes the transmission of nociceptive information to the brain. Descartes' early model of nociception describes a simple path from transduction to perception of the painful stimulus. However, experience tells us that the relationship between injury and perception of pain is unpredictable and non-linear. We know now that this is because *modulation* of nociception can occur at all levels of the conducting system, reducing or enhancing our perception of pain. Moreover, the structure and function of the conducting system itself can change dynamically in response to input, a phenomenon known as *plasticity*.

This chapter describes the anatomy, physiology and pathophysiology of pain, under the following headings:

- Transduction
- Transmission
- Perception
- Modulation
- Plasticity
- Mechanisms of neuropathic pain.

Transduction

Conversion of a painful stimulus to a pain signal (transduction) takes place at the pain receptor, or *nociceptor*. Peripheral nociceptors are the free nerve endings of finely myelinated Aδ- and unmyelinated C-fibres, the character-istics of which are shown in Figures 2.1 and 2.2.

Compared with sensitive, low-threshold mechanoreceptors and thermo-receptors responsible for touch and temperature sensation, nociceptors have a relatively high activation threshold and respond only to intense, noxious stimuli. Both C and Aδ nociceptors are *polymodal*, responding to mechani-cal and thermal noxious stimuli, as well as various chemicals released in response to tissue injury and inflammation (*see* Figure 2.3). In addition, myelinated Aδ nociceptors signal the sharp pain from acute mechanical or thermal injury [1].

Visceral pain is subserved by a similar population of Aδ- and C-fibres, trav-elling with autonomic afferents. Visceral nociceptors respond to distension, ischaemia and inflammation, but not to cutting and thermal damage.

Transmission

Primary afferent conduction

Transduction at the nociceptor generates an action potential, which is propagated along the axon of the primary afferent neuron. Primary afferent cell bodies lie in the dorsal root ganglia or trigeminal ganglion, and their central processes enter the dorsal horn of the spinal cord via the dorsal roots.

Anatomy of the dorsal horn

The spinal cord in cross-section consists of an 'H' shape of grey matter (cell bodies) surrounded by white matter (myelinated axons). The 'H' shape consists of paired ventral and dorsal horns.

The dorsal horn is the relay point for sensory information converging from the periphery. Rexed [2] subdivided the grey matter of the dorsal horn into distinct laminae, based on cytoarchitecture (*see* Figure 2.4).

C-fibres terminate in lamina II, the substantia gelatinosa. Aδ-fibres terminate primarily in lamina I, but some project more deeply to terminate

Figure 2.1 Characteristics of primary afferent pain fibres

Fibre type	Aδ	C
Diameter	2–5 µm	< 2 µm
Conduction velocity	5–15 m/sec	0.5–2 m/sec
Type of pain subserved	'Fast', pinprick, well localized	'Slow', diffuse, dull, aching
Distribution of nociceptors	Skin, muscle, joints	Most tissues

Figure 2.2 Characteristics of primary afferent fibres of the nervous system

A. Characteristics of primary afferent pain fibres

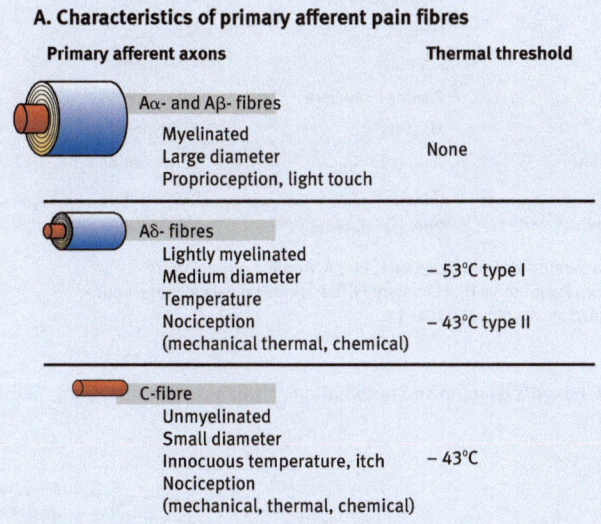

Primary afferent axons

Thermal threshold

Aα- and Aβ- fibres
Myelinated
Large diameter
Proprioception, light touch

None

Aδ- fibres
Lightly myelinated
Medium diameter
Temperature
Nociception
(mechanical thermal, chemical)

− 53°C type I

− 43°C type II

C-fibre
Unmyelinated
Small diameter
Innocuous temperature, itch
Nociception
(mechanical, thermal, chemical)

− 43°C

B. Conduction velocity, fibre type and pain

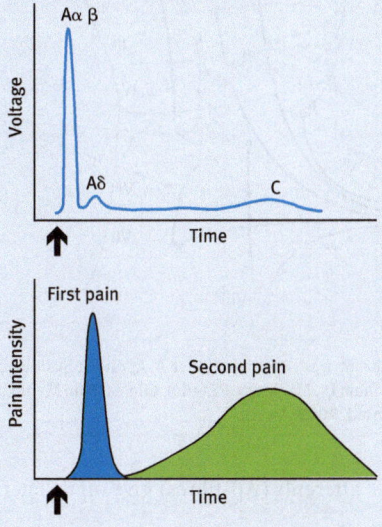

Figure 2.3 Endogenous molecules activating nociceptors

Substance	Source	Effect on nociceptors
Potassium	Damaged cells	Activation
Protons	Hypoxic cells	Activation
Serotonin	Platelets	Activation
Bradykinin	Plasma kininogen	Activation
Histamine	Mast cells	Activation
Prostaglandin	Damaged cells	Sensitization
Leukotrienes	Damaged cells	Sensitization
Substance P	Primary afferents	Sensitization

Adapted with permission from Beaulieu P, Rice A. Applied physiology of
nociception. In: Rowbotham DJ, Macintyre PE (eds). Clinical Pain Management –
Acute Pain. London: Arnold, 2003: 4–16.

Figure 2.4 Rexed's laminae and termination of primary afferent neurons in the
dorsal horn

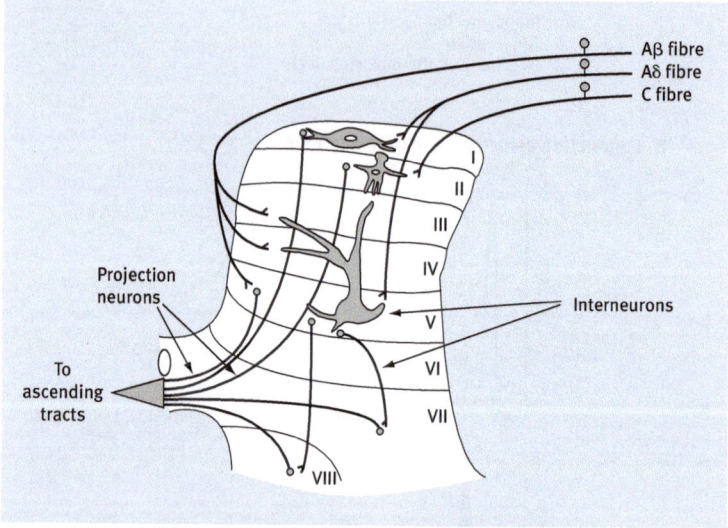

Reproduced with permission from Beaulieu P, Rice A. Applied physiology of
nociception. In: Rowbotham DJ, Macintyre PE (eds). Clinical Pain Management –
Acute Pain. London: Arnold, 2003: 4–16.

in lamina V. Tactile afferents (Aβ-fibres) give off collaterals that terminate
in laminae III–V.

Primary afferent fibres synapse in the dorsal horn with second-order
neurons, of which there are three main types: projection neurons, responsible

for onward transmission to higher centres, and excitatory and inhibitory interneurons.

Physiologically, second-order neurons can be divided into three discrete types:

1. Nociceptive specific (NS) – responding exclusively to noxious stimuli.
2. Low threshold (LT) – responding to non-noxious input.
3. Wide dynamic range (WDR) – responding to a range of stimuli, receiving converging inputs from multiple afferent inputs.

Visceral nociceptive input is not as well defined, because fewer nociceptors activate a larger number of second-order spinal neurons. Visceral afferents terminate in laminae I and V and, by converging with somatic inputs at these levels, may account for referred pain.

Neurotransmitters at the dorsal horn

A variety of neurotransmitters is involved in *excitatory* nociceptive transmission at the dorsal horn, primarily the amino acids *glutamate* and *aspartate*. These activate the AMPA (α-amino-3-hydroxy-5-methyl-4-isoxazolepropionate) subtype of glutamate receptor, and have an indirect effect on the *NMDA* (*N*-methyl-D-aspartate) receptor. Activation of the NMDA receptor, thought to play a pivotal role in mediating spinal hyperalgesia, is complex and requires sustained C-fibre activity. *Neuropeptides* such as substance P and CGRP (calcitonin gene-related peptide) probably facilitate the excitatory amino acids. Metabotropic (operating by signal transduction rather than by ion channel activity) glutamate receptors, or *mGluRs*, have a role in synaptic plasticity, as well as modulation of activity at other receptors. (See below for a description of inhibitory neurotransmitters modulating the nociception at the dorsal horn.)

Ascending tracts

Approximately 90% of second-order neurons in the dorsal horn decussate to the contralateral side of the spinal cord before ascending in the spinothalamic and spinoreticular tracts.

The *spinothalamic tract* originates from Aδ neurons in laminae I and V of the dorsal horn and ascends anterolaterally in the white matter of the cord. The *lateral spinothalamic tract (neospinothalamic)* ascends directly to the ventral, posterior, lateral nucleus of the thalamus. It subserves the sensory-discriminative aspect of pain perception.

The phylogenetically older *medial spinothalamic tract (paleospinothalamic)* is a polysynaptic pathway which sends collaterals to the periaqueductal grey matter (PAG), hypothalamus and reticular system in the midbrain, and then to the medial thalamus. This tract is thought to be responsible for mediating the autonomic and unpleasant emotional component of the pain experience.

Both spinothalamic tracts then relay via tertiary afferents to higher structures within the brain (*see* Figure 2.5).

Figure 2.5 Ascending pathways: spinothalamic tracts

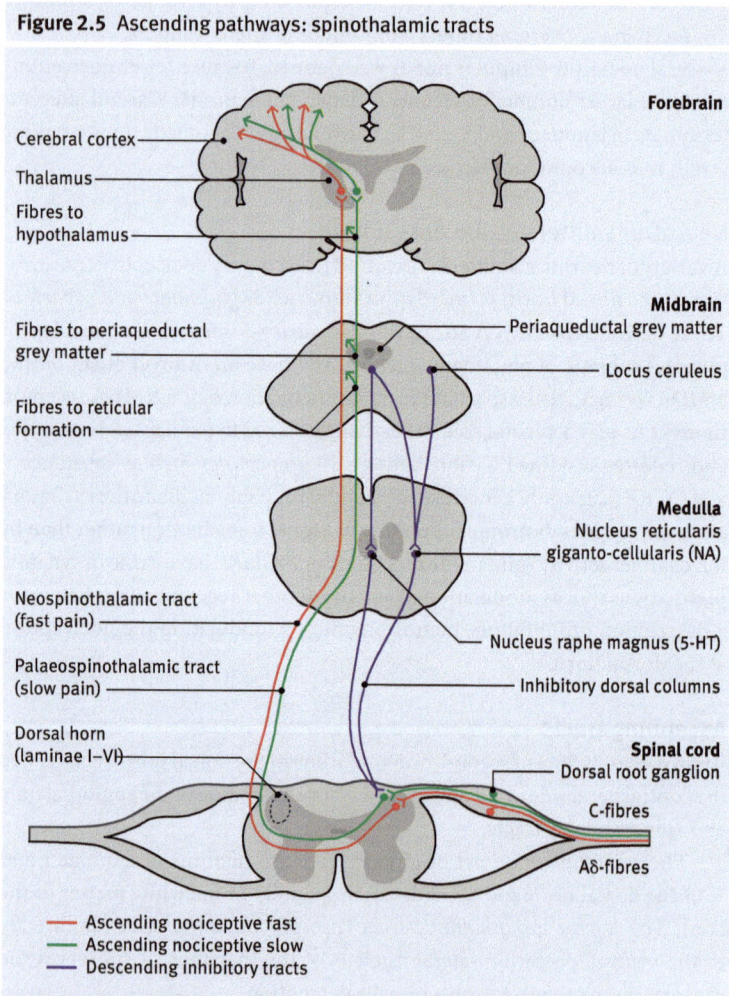

See Modulation (this chapter) for further discussion of descending inhibition.
Reproduced with permission from Serpell M. Anatomy, physiology and pharmacology of pain. Anaesth Intens Care Med 2005; 6:7–10.
NA, norepinephrine (noradrenaline); 5-HT, 5-hydroxytryptamine.

The *spinoreticular tract* is phylogenetically ancient. It originates from neurons in the deeper laminae VII and VIII, and terminates in the reticular formation of the medulla and pons. From there, information is relayed to the thalamus and hypothalamus, with diffuse projections to the whole cerebral cortex. The spinoreticular system subserves the diffuse, emotionally unpleasant component of pain.

Laminae I and V neurons also project to the *spinomesencephalic tract*, terminating in the roof of the midbrain (superior colliculus), and projecting to the mesencephalic PAG. The spinomesencephalic tract is not thought to be vital for pain perception, but modulates nociception, possibly through endogenous opioids and descending inhibitory pathways [3].

The *parabrachial* pathway receives spinal input primarily from lamina I, and projects to the hypothalamus, amygdala and a portion of the thalamus subserving visceral sensory activity. Thus, the parabrachial pathway provides a substrate for integration of nociceptive activity with general visceral (homeostatic) afferent activity [4].

Perception

Pain is a complex experience, incorporating both sensory–discriminative and affective–motivational components. Functional magnetic resonance imaging (fMRI) and positron emission tomography (PET) techniques have given us insight into which regions of the brain are involved in pain perception (*see* Figure 2.6).

The primary and secondary somatosensory cortexes are associated with sensory and discriminative aspects of nociception, while the deeper limbic structures are associated with the affective–motivational components of the pain experience [5]. The anterior cingulate cortex (ACC) in particular is thought to play an important role in the emotional and aversive component of pain.

Modulation

It is common experience that pain does not necessarily follow injury – a twisted ankle might not be noticed until after the marathon has been run, or a battlefield injury might be painless until the soldier reaches a place of safety. This implies that modulation of the pain signal must occur at some point along the pathway.

The dorsal horn is the major interface between the peripheral and central nervous systems, and most of the physiological modulation that we know about takes place here. There are four main mechanisms for modulation at the dorsal horn:

1. Endogenous opioids.

Figure 2.6 Schematic representation of subcortical structures and cerebral cortical structures involved in processing pain

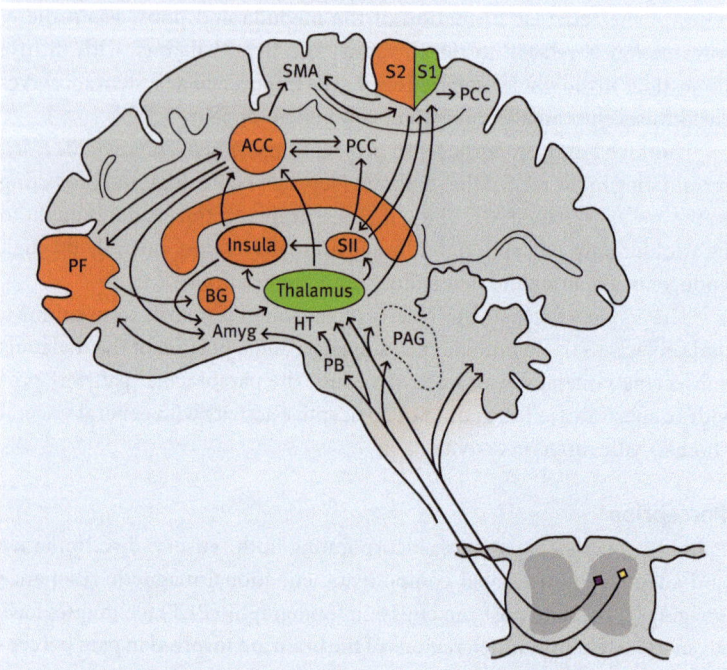

ACC, anterior cingulate cortex; Amyg, amygdala; BG, basal ganglia; HT, hypothalamus; PAG, periaqueductal grey; PB, parabrachial nucleus of the dorsolateral pons; PCC, posterior cingulate cortex; PF, prefrontal cortex; PPC, posterior parietal complex; SI and SII, first and second somatosensory cortical areas; SMA, supplementary motor area.
Reproduced with permission from Bushnell M, Apkarin A. Representation of pain in the brain. In: McMahon S, Koltzenburg M (eds). Wall and Melzack's Textbook of Pain. Edinburgh: Churchill Livingstone, 2006.

2. Segmental (local) inhibition.

3. 'Gate control' (modulation by non-nociceptive input).

4. Descending inhibition from higher centres.

Endogenous opioids

There are three main classes of endogenous opioids, the *endorphins*, *dynorphins* and *enkephalins*. Of these, the endorphins and enkephalins are thought to play an important role in modulating nociception at the dorsal horn. Opioid receptors (delta [δ], kappa [κ], and mu [μ]) are found mainly in laminae I and II (substantia gelatinosa) of the dorsal horn (*see* Figure 2.7).

Figure 2.7 Characteristics of opioid receptors at the dorsal horn

Type of receptor	μ	δ	κ
Prevalence in spinal cord (%)	70	24	6
Endogenous ligand*	Endomorphin-7 Endorphin-31	Enkephalin-5 Endorphin-31	Dynorphin-17
Exogenous ligand	Morphine	None	Enadoline
Action of ligand	Opens K+	Opens K+	Closes Ca2+
Analgesia	Good	Good	Poor
Primary CNS effect	Respiratory depression	Respiratory stimulation	Psychomimetic
Effect on gut	Constipation	–	–
Cholecytokinin effect at receptor	Inhibits	None	None

*Number indicates number of amino acids that form the compound.

The principal action of endogenous opioids at these receptors is to produce pre-synaptic inhibition at the synapse between primary afferent and second-order neurons. The effect is short-lived.

Segmental inhibition

Distinct from descending inhibitory pathways, local inhibition is mediated at the dorsal horn by a variety of inhibitory neurotransmitters. The role of the inhibitory amino acids gamma-aminobutyric acid (GABA) and glycine is well established, but many other neurotransmitters and receptors have been studied (*see* Figure 2.8).

Gate control theory

Gate control theory is a model proposed by Melzack and Wall [6] in 1965, whereby activity from non-nociceptive Aβ afferents inhibits onward transmission of nociceptive signals from Aδ and C afferents. An inhibitory interneuron acts as a physiological 'gate', which is closed by Aβ-afferent activity (*see* Figure 2.9). The theory is the basis for neuromodulation techniques such as TENS (transcutaneous electrical nerve stimulation) and spinal cord stimulation.

Descending inhibition

Psychological factors, such as arousal and attention, have a well-established effect on pain perception. We are beginning to identify descending pathways and networks that could play a part in supraspinal inhibition of nociceptive transmission.

Figure 2.8 Neurotransmitters modulating nociception at the dorsal horn

Neurotransmitter	Receptor type	Effect on nociception
GABA	GABA-A, GABA-B	Inhibits
Glycine		Inhibits
Enkephalins	Opioid receptors ($\delta > \kappa$, μ)	Inhibits
β-Endorphins	Opioid receptors ($\mu > \delta$, κ)	Inhibits
Cannabinoids	CB_1	Inhibits
Nitric oxide	(via cGMP increase)	Excitatory
CCK	CCK_B	Inhibits opioid receptor
5-HT (serotonin)	$5HT_1$	Inhibits
Norepinephrine (noradrenaline)	α_2	Inhibits
Galanin	GAL	Inhibits

GABA, gamma-aminobutyric acid; CCK, cholecystokinin.
Adapted with permission from Beaulieu P, Rice A. Applied physiology of nociception. In: Rowbotham DJ, Macintyre PE (eds). Clinical Pain Management – Acute Pain. London: Arnold, 2003: 4–16.

Figure 2.9 Gate control theory

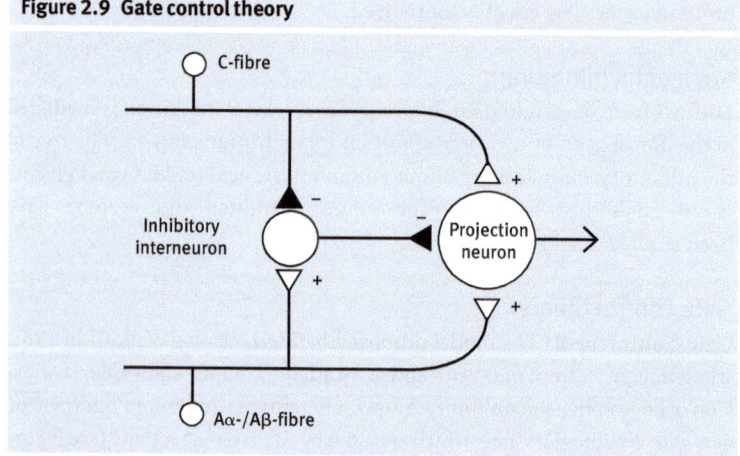

Reproduced with permission from Beaulieu P, Rice A. Applied physiology of nociception. In: Rowbotham DJ, Macintyre PE (eds). Clinical Pain Management – Acute Pain. London: Arnold, 2003: 4–16.

Two main relay areas have been identified, in the midbrain *periaqueductal grey matter* and the *rostral ventromedial medulla* (RVM). The PAG–RVM network receives inputs from the *limbic system*, providing a mechanism by which emotional factors might influence pain perception. Descending fibres make inhibitory connections at laminae I, II and V of the dorsal horn. The primary neurotransmitters in these descending pathways are serotonin (5-HT) and norepinephrine (noradrenaline) – a possible reason for the analgesic efficacy of tricyclic antidepressants and tramadol.

In addition, the PAG–RVM system is the main central site of action of opioids. Morphine injected directly to this region has a greater analgesic effect than at any other site in the CNS. However, the relative importance of brain versus spinal opioid receptors in modulating nociception is not known [3].

Plasticity

The nervous system is not hard-wired. Neurons can change their structure and function in response to certain inputs or changes in their environment, a phenomenon known as *plasticity*. Plasticity is seen at all levels of the nociceptive system, from peripheral nociceptors to the cerebral cortex. Changes can occur following nerve injury, or simply in response to sustained nociceptive input. These changes can be short-lived or permanent. The molecular processes and synaptic changes observed in chronic pain states are thought to be similar to those changes underlying normal physiological processes such as learning and memory [7]. Plasticity plays an important part in the central sensitization observed in neuropathic pain.

Following tissue injury, skin surrounding the injured area becomes more sensitive to painful stimuli, a phenomenon known as *hyperalgesia*. Hyperalgesia following tissue injury appears to have two components: local sensitization of primary afferent nociceptors by inflammatory mediators produces *primary hyperalgesia*, with an attendant local flare reaction. A later area of *secondary hyperalgesia* then develops in uninjured skin surrounding the inflamed area. Local anaesthetic nerve block proximal to the injured skin prevents development of secondary hyperalgesia, demonstrating that secondary hyperalgesia is a centrally mediated phenomenon (*see* Figure 2.10).

A well-studied example of central plasticity is that of activation-dependent plasticity in dorsal horn neurons – the phenomenon of 'wind-up', whereby repeated activation of C-fibre nociceptors by an intense or sustained noxious stimulus can increase the duration of the excitatory response by dorsal horn neurons. Wind-up is transient, terminating with cessation of the stimulus. Longer-term potentiation has been demonstrated, mediated by NMDA-receptor activation.

Intense nociceptive input also induces *transcriptional changes* at the dorsal horn. Noxious stimulation and inflammation can produce alterations in gene expression that lead to loss of inhibitory interneurons, contributing

Figure 2.10 Proximal nerve block prevents the development of secondary hyperalgesia

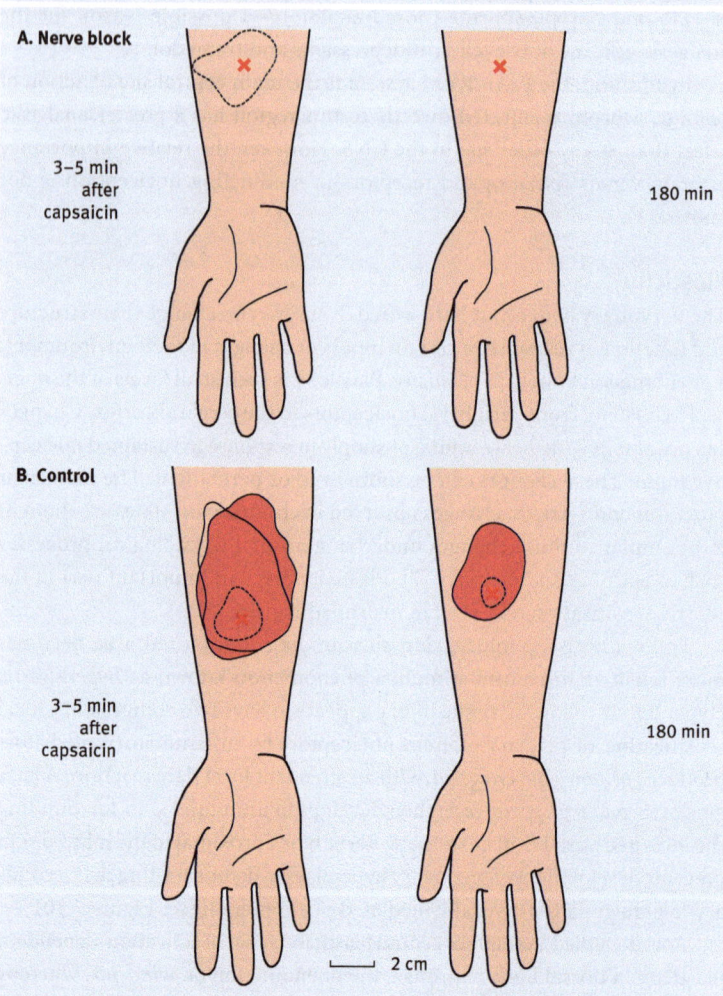

A After blockade of the lateral antebrachial nerve with 1% xylocaine, capsaicin (100 µg in 10 µL) was injected into the anaesthetic skin. A flare (dashed line) developed within 5 min. No hyperalgesia was present 180 min after the capsaicin injection when the local anaesthetic block had recovered. **B** On the control arm, normal flare and hyperalgesia to stroking (dotted line) and punctate (solid line, shaded) stimuli developed within 5 min. Hyperalgesia to punctate stimuli was still present 180 min after the capsaicin injection. Reproduced with permission from LaMotte RH, Shain CN, Simone DA, Tsai EF. Neurogenic hyperalgesia: psychophysical studies of underlying mechanisms. J Neurophysiol 1991; 66:190–211.

to central sensitization. These activity-dependent transcriptional changes are also observed peripherally.

Functional brain imaging techniques have demonstrated rapid and persistent reorganization of cortical somatosensory maps following limb amputation. The territory that once represented the amputated limb no longer receives afferent input, and adjacent somatosensory representation areas expand to fill the vacant space (*see* Figure 2.11). There appears to be a correlation between degree of cortical reorganization and intensity of phantom limb pain. Imaging studies in patients with fibromyalgia and chronic back pain have also demonstrated cortical reorganization.

Mechanisms of neuropathic pain

Neuropathic pain is a pathological pain, defined by the IASP as 'pain initiated or caused by a primary lesion or dysfunction in the nervous system' [8]. Any disease process that causes injury to the nervous system, from diabetic neuropathy in the periphery to thalamic stroke centrally, can give rise to neuropathic pain.

Figure 2.11 Schematic diagram illustrating the shift in area of somatosensory representation of the lip following upper limb amputation

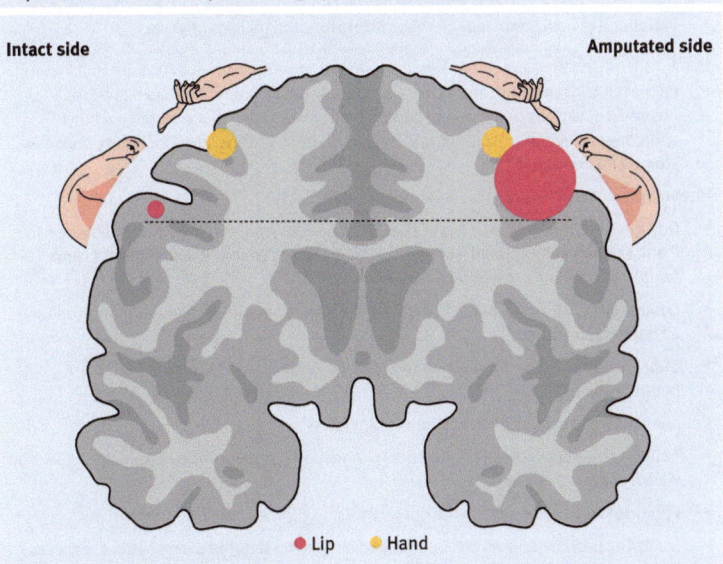

Intact side   Amputated side

● Lip   ● Hand

Adapted from Knecht S, Henningsen H, Elbert T, et al. Reorganizational and perceptional changes after amputation. Brain 1996; 119(Pt 4):1213–19.

The response of the CNS to injury produces the symptoms and signs characteristic of neuropathic pain, generally reflecting a state of increased excitation and decreased inhibition throughout the pain-conducting system.

Peripheral changes following nerve injury are summarized in Figure 2.12. Peripheral changes can also result in *central sensitization* – enhanced transmission of, and increased sensitivity to, nociceptive inputs at the dorsal horn. Figure 2.13 summarizes changes at the dorsal horn thought to mediate central sensitization.

The exact relationship between these changes and the symptoms and signs characteristic of neuropathic pain is unclear, though in some cases a relationship seems likely. For example, following peripheral nerve injury,

Figure 2.12 Peripheral changes in response to nerve injury

CNS response to injury – peripheral changes

Sensitization of primary afferent nociceptor terminals

- Following nerve injury, antidromic conduction of action potentials can lead to release of neuropeptides, which sensitize nerve terminals of both injured and adjacent non-injured fibres
- Sensitization results in a lower activation threshold, increased response to a given stimulus and spontaneous discharges
- Peripheral sensitization may be responsible for primary hyperalgesia

Ectopic discharges

- Increased concentration and activity of sodium and calcium channels has been observed at various points along neurons following nerve injury: this can result in spontaneous ectopic discharge and hyperactivity at various sites, including proximal stump and neuromas

Phenotypic switch in expression of neuropeptides

- Down-regulation in expression of specific neurotransmitters, including substance P and calcium gene-related peptide, has been observed in primary afferent C- and Aδ-fibres following peripheral nerve injury
- Concurrently, Aβ-fibres begin to express these neuropeptides, a phenomenon known as phenotypic switch
- Subsequent low-threshold activation of Aβ-fibres may lead to release of these neurotransmitters

Coupling between sympathetic and sensory nervous systems

- Coupling may occur by direct electrical connection (ephapse) or by chemical connection via adrenergic receptors
- Ephapses have been seen in the dorsal root ganglion and the periphery
- Following partial nerve injury, injured and adjacent uninjured axons begin to express α-adrenoceptors (up-regulated in axon and dorsal root ganglion). These changes might explain the enhanced sensitivity to catecholamines observed in some patients with sympathetically maintained pain

Figure 2.13 Spinal cord dorsal horn changes mediating central sensitization

CNS response to injury – central sensitization

Spinal reorganization

- Normally, Aδ- and C-fibres that are responsible for nociceptive transmission terminate on the superficial laminae I and II of the dorsal horn, while large myelinated non-nociceptive fibres (Aβ) terminate in laminae III and IV

- Following peripheral nerve injury, Aβ-fibres have been shown to form connections on to lamina II, i.e. fibres that convey non-nociceptive information synapse with cells in the dorsal horn that deal specifically with nociception

- This is a possible explanation for the phenomenon of mechanical allodynia

Depression of inhibitory synapses at the dorsal horn (disinhibition)

- This occurs via a decrease in the amount of the inhibitory neurotransmitter, gamma-aminobutyric acid (GABA) in the dorsal horn, and down-regulation of GABA receptors post-synaptically

- Opioid receptors are also down-regulated

Ectopic activity

- Excitatory synapses in the dorsal horn may be facilitated

- Spontaneous discharges from dorsal horn cells have been observed following dorsal rhizotomy (neurosurgical transection of nerve roots)

Activation-dependent plasticity in dorsal horn neurons – 'wind-up' phenomenon

- Repeated activation of C-fibre nociceptors by an intense or sustained noxious stimulus can increase the duration of the excitatory response by dorsal horn neurons.

Activation of wide dynamic range (WDR) neurons

- Spinal WDR neurons have small receptive zones for non-noxious stimuli that are surrounded by, and overlap with, a larger receptive field for noxious stimuli

- Overlap of the fields may explain referred pain and the spread of sensory dysfunction proximal and distal to a nerve injury

Aβ-fibres conveying non-nociceptive information synapse with nociceptive neurons in lamina II of the dorsal horn. This is likely to be related to the phenomenon of mechanical allodynia, or pain produced in response to a normally non-noxious stimulus.

References

1. Meyer R, Ringkamp M, Campbell J, Raja S. Peripheral mechanisms of cutaneous nociception. In: McMahon S, Koltzenburg M (eds). Wall and Melzack's Textbook of Pain. Edinburgh: Churchill Livingstone, 2006.
2. Rexed B. The cytoarchitectonic organisation of the spinal cord of cat. J Comparative Neurol 1952; 96: 415–95.
3. Beaulieu P, Rice A. Applied physiology of nociception. In: Rowbotham DJ, Macintyre PE (eds). Clinical Pain Management – Acute Pain. London: Arnold, 2003: 4–16.
4. Dostrovsky J, Craig A. Ascending projection systems. In: McMahon S, Koltzenburg M (eds). Wall and Melzack's Textbook of Pain. Edinburgh: Churchill Livingstone, 2006.

5. Bushnell M, Apkarin A. Representation of pain in the brain. In: McMahon S, Koltzenburg M (eds). Wall and Melzack's Textbook of Pain. Edinburgh: Churchill Livingstone, 2006.
6. Wall P, Melzack R. Pain mechanisms: a new theory. Science 1965; 150:171–9.
7. Woolf C, Salter M. Plasticity and pain: role of the dorsal horn. In: McMahon S, Koltzenburg M (eds). Wall and Melzack's Textbook of Pain. Edinburgh: Churchill Livingstone, 2006.
8. Merskey H, Bogduk N (eds). Classification of Chronic Pain: Descriptions of Chronic Pain Syndromes and Definitions of Pain Terms, 2nd edn. IASP Task Force on Taxonomy. Seattle, WA: IASP Press, 1994.

Chapter 3

Patient evaluation

The key to successful management of pain in any patient is accurate assessment. For one of the most universal symptoms in medicine this is a surprisingly (but not unexpectedly) difficult task. Chronic painful conditions are present in virtually all medical specialties and the impact of pain on the patient can occur on several levels. This breadth of understanding means that a clinician may often need to use assessment skills developed from other specialities such as orthopaedics and psychology in the same pain patient.

Due to its complexity it took medicine almost 2000 years to produce a universally agreed definition of pain [1]. Patients may suffer completely different experiences which can all be described as painful. Patients may undergo the same pain experiences (such as hernia surgery or suffering osteoarthritis of the hip) and yet report wildly differing pain intensity. Pain is not only a sensory phenomenon but also incorporates an affective and cognitive experience with many of the higher levels of the nervous system involved. This understanding of pain based predominantly on research in the musculoskeleletal field [2] has led to pain being viewed as a *biopsychosocial phenomenon* (*see* Figure 3.1).

Due to the subjective nature of pain, it is better to go with the maxim of 'pain is what the patient says it is' rather than undertaking elaborate measures to prove whether a patient has 'genuine' pain. For chronic pain with no obvious cause, this may lead to attempts at diagnosis but it is not an invitation for widespread and detailed investigations. Rather it is an understanding that, while illness behaviour and psychological distress are common in some chronic pain conditions, it is rare for a patient to fabricate their painful symptoms completely.

At a basic level many approaches have been used to evaluate pain as a single phenomenon. One-dimensional pain scales have proved to be very useful in the measurement of acute pain, leading to pain being viewed as a fifth vital sign [3].

Figure 3.1 Modified biopsychosocial model

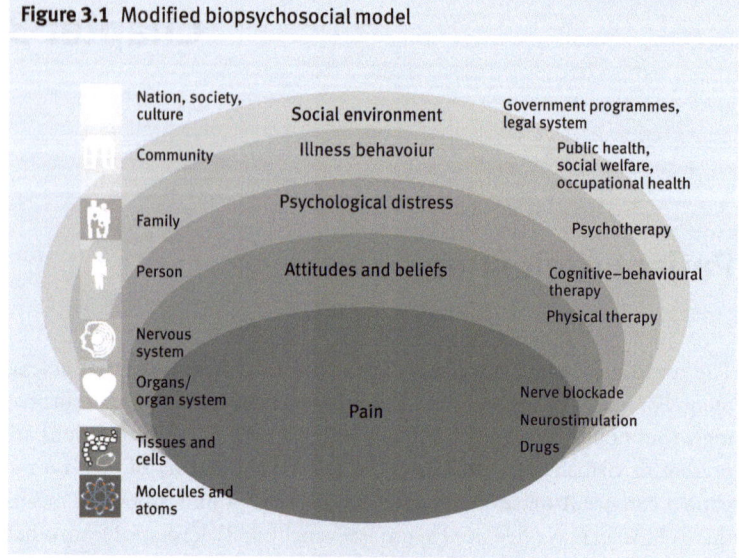

Reproduced with permission from NHS Quality Improvement Scotland.
Management of chronic pain in adults. Best practice statement – February 2006.
Edinburgh: NHS Quality Improvement Scotland, 2006.

Categorical scales use words such as none, mild, moderate or severe and allocate them a numerical ranking (0 = none, 3 = severe). This has been adapted for children with the so-called FACES pain scale (*see* Figure 3.2).

Visual analogue scales (VAS) produce a line between no and worst possible pain, or alternatively may assess the benefit of an analgesic intervention by a line between no pain relief and complete pain relief; patients are asked to place a mark corresponding to their experience.

Figure 3.2 Wong–Baker FACES Pain Rating Scale

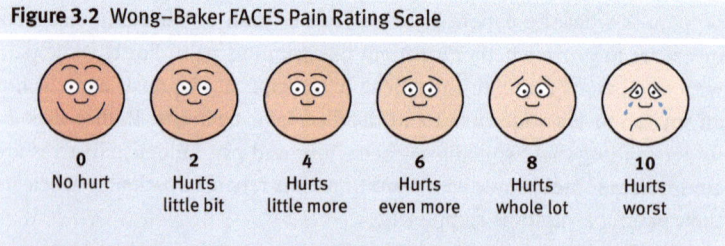

Point to each face using the words to describe the pain intensity. Ask the child to choose face that best describes own pain and record the appropriate number.

From Hockenberry MJ, Wilson D, Winkelstein ML. Wong's Essentials of Pediatric Nursing, 7th edn. St Louis, MO: Mosby, Inc., 2005:1259. Used with permission. Copyright, Mosby.

Numerical scales work on a similar basis with patients being asked to rate their pain out of 10, with 0 being pain free and 10 being 'worst possible' pain.

Intrapatient reliability within these scales is good and they are simple to use. Their limitations occur when the pain that patients experience is more complex or they have more than one pain. There is often a tendency for patients to avoid the extremes of measurement, which results in a bias towards a midline value.

Chronic pain measurement is much more complex and this is reflected by the number of measurement scales produced and their multidimensional nature. These are time-consuming, often difficult for the patient to understand and more likely to be used on a research basis. Multiple questionnaires have been proposed, none of which have become the gold standard for chronic pain measures. The widely used McGill Pain Questionnaire looks at the sensory and affective components of pain as well as evaluating intensity. Other more patient-friendly scales have also been developed, such as the Short-Form McGill Pain Questionnaire or the Brief Pain Inventory.

At a research level, psychophysical tests such as quantitative sensory testing have been seen as an attempt to provide more objective measures of chronic pain assessment for disorders such as neuropathic pain. This involves measuring various pain thresholds in response to stimuli such as heat or pressure. Although extensively investigated at a research level, this technique has yet to be transferred into mainstream clinical practice.

Practical assessment

As with any initial assessment a full history and systemic enquiry are mandatory (*see* Figure 3.3). Any concerns elicited in a thorough systemic inquiry need to be investigated or referred to an appropriate physician. It is important to have some idea of the quality of the pain itself, as well as its interactions, and to bear in mind that *not all pains are the same*.

Nociceptive pain ('normal' pain) arises from mechanical, chemical or thermal stimulation of nociceptors (e.g. after surgery, trauma or associated with degenerative processes such as osteoarthritis). It may be somatic or visceral. It can present with a wide variety of symptoms (*see* Figure 3.4). Generally most acute and cancer pain will have some form of nociceptive basis but it is important to realize that pain may persist long after the nociceptive process has ended and that other factors, e.g. psychosocial features, may need to be considered.

Neuropathic pain is initiated or caused by a primary lesion or dysfunction in the nervous system to the peripheral or central nervous system (i.e. in conditions such as painful diabetic neuropathy or spinal cord injury).

Figure 3.3 Specific questions about a patient's pain

- Site
- Radiation
- Quality (dull, sharp, throbbing, etc.)
- Severity
- Duration
- Frequency
- Periodicity
- Precipitating factors
- Relieving factors
- Associated phenomena (nausea, sweating, muscle spasm, etc.)
- Therapies (drugs, interventions, alternative therapy)

Figure 3.4 Features of nociceptive ('normal') pain

Somatic nociceptive pain

- Well-localized site with dermatomal radiation
- Variable character, which may range from aching to sharp
- May be constant but have 'incident' breakthroughs, e.g. on movement
- Few autonomic associations

Visceral nociceptive pain

- Often vague distribution with a diffuse radiation
- Dull, crampy character
- Colicky and periodic
- Often associated with autonomic symptoms

It has quite different clinical features from nociceptive pain (*see* Figure 3.5). It is less well localized and often described as burning or shooting. It can occur in areas that are numb and where there is no tissue damage.

The Neuropathic Pain Scale (NPS) [4] was developed to quantify the components of neuropathic pain so that its progression or response to treatment could be followed over time. The Leeds Assessment of Neuropathic Symptoms and Signs (LANSS) [5] was developed as a screening tool to help differentiate neuropathic pain from nociceptive pain in a more standardized way (*see* Figure 3.6).

Psychosocial features have been shown to be predictors of the incidence and duration of chronic pain. It is important to realize that this does not imply that the pain has a psychological basis, only that psychological and social factors may be important drivers in the severity and maintenance of pain, amount of functional impairment and degree of responsiveness to treatment. When pain lasts longer than 3 months or beyond the time when

Figure 3.5 Features of neuropathic pain

- May be unaccompanied by ongoing tissue damage and also occur in an area of sensory loss

- May be burning or lancinating in nature. Dysaesthesia (unpleasant abnormal sensations, such as 'pins and needles') can occur

- May be greater than expected pain in response to a painful stimulus (hyperalgesia), or pain that increases with a repetitive stimulus (hyperpathia). Light touch may produce neuropathic pain (allodynia)

Figure 3.6 Screening questions from the Leeds Assessment of Neuropathic Symptoms and Signs (LANSS)

- Would you describe your pain as strange unpleasant sensations in your skin? (e.g. pricking, tingling, pins and needles) – Yes/No

- Does the skin in the painful areas look different to normal? (e.g. mottled, more red/pink than usual) – Yes/No

- Is the skin in the affected area abnormally sensitive to touch? (e.g. unpleasant sensations if lightly stroked, painful to wear tight clothes) – Yes/No

- Does your pain come on suddenly in bursts for no apparent reason when you are still? (e.g. like electric shocks, 'bursting' or 'jumping' sensations) – Yes/No

- Do you feel that skin temperature in the painful area has changed (e.g. hot, burning) – Yes/No

- Does stroking the affected area of skin with a piece of cotton wool produce an unpleasant painful sensation? – Yes/No

- Does touching the affected area of skin with a sharp needle feel sharper or duller when compared with an area of normal skin? – Yes/No

A positive response to each question adds a varying numerical score, which, if it adds up to greater than 12 out of 24, is highly suggestive of neuropathic pain.
Based on information from Bennett M. The LANSS Pain Scale: the Leeds assessment of neuropathic symptoms and signs. Pain 2001; 92:147–57.

an acute injury would be expected to have healed, the patient's presentation becomes more complex. There may be more psychological features, including complaints of poor or non-refreshing sleep, tiredness, depression and poor concentration. Baseline assessment of functional ability can provide more objective and verifiable information about a patient's quality of life and ability to participate in normal life activities.

An assessment of the relative contributions and dynamics of family and personal relationships, financial situation, employment record, past pain experiences and personality should be made. A patient's fear of pain, interpretation of what the pain means and its likely effects have become important targets of psychological therapy.

A number of psychosocial 'yellow flags' have been found to be useful in predicting failure to return to work after back injury, and also prove useful in predicting which patients are more likely to develop prolonged pain in other situations (*see* Figure 3.7) [6].

It is essential also to elicit any history of depression or other psychopathology that may affect the perception of pain. Past or current physical, sexual or emotional abuse may be important in some chronic pain states. Suicidal ideation should be assessed where indicated. Any history of chemical dependency in both the patient and family members should be elicited because this can have an impact on therapy. Patients should be carefully screened for risk of medication diversion or abuse. The behaviours shown in Figure 3.8 suggest relative contraindications to opioid use in non-malignant pain. With these patients, referral to a pain or addiction specialist is advisable.

The CAGE questionnaire, which asks specific questions about cutting down drinking, anger, guilt or early morning drinking, is a useful tool for brief alcohol screening of the patient [7].

Figure 3.7 Psychosocial features associated with chronic back pain ('yellow flags')

1 Presence of a belief that the pain is harmful or potentially severely disabling

2 Fear-avoidance behaviour (avoiding a movement or activity because of a misplaced anticipation of pain) and reduced activity levels

3 Tendency to low mood and withdrawal from social interaction

4 An expectation that passive treatments rather than active participation will help

5 High degrees of health anxiety and illness behaviour

6 Family reinforcement (e.g. a spouse who is overprotective)

7 Employment issues (e.g. both low-intensity and high-intensity work)

8 Litigation (e.g. a work accident claim)

Adapted from Kendall NAS, Linton SJ, Main CJ. Guide to assessing psychosocial yellow flags in acute low back pain: risk factors for long-term disability and work loss. Wellington, NZ: Accident Rehabilitation & Compensation Insurance Corporation of New Zealand, and the National Health Committee, Ministry of Health, 1997.

Figure 3.8 Risk factors for opiate prescription in non-malignant pain

- History of substance abuse or prior prescription drug misuse
- Unsanctioned dose escalations on several occasions
- Non-adherence to other recommendations for pain therapy
- Unwillingness or inability to comply with treatment plan
- Social instability
- Unwillingness to adjust at-risk activities resulting in serious re-injury requiring additional opiate prescriptions

Acute pain

Most acute pain is a single phenomenon and nociceptive in nature. Assessment is routinely done by unidimensional scales, e.g. VAS. Problems occur when an acute neuropathic pain also occurs or when a chronic pain patient with significant complexity and psychosocial factors presents with an acute pain problem. Liaison between both acute and chronic pain services is essential.

Cancer pain

Good cancer pain assessment incorporates all the key features of pain assessment. The severity and quality of the pain, e.g. nociceptive, neuropathic, need to be assessed. Associated symptoms of both the cancer and the therapy, e.g. constipation, sedation, inform the options available. As well as eliciting psychosocial features, e.g. depression, some assessment of spiritual pain is useful in relieving patient anxiety. There are specific concerns in relation to cancer therapy, e.g. vincristine-induced neuropathy, which may need to be assessed. Liaison with palliative care services is essential. As well as initiating treatment, palliative care support will allow the patient both the time and the space to raise issues in relation to disease progression.

Chronic pain

Chronic pain frequently involves the musculoskeletal system and the nervous system. These areas should be examined more carefully and with attention to possible clinical diagnosis of pain relative to the patient's history.

Musculoskeletal system

Skeletal muscle pain is a common cause of chronic pain. Chronic back pain is a frequent cause of referral. It is important to recognize signs of significant pathology ('red flags') (*see* Figure 3.9).

Figure 3.9 Indicators of serious pathology in back pain ('red flags')

1 Age under 20 or over 55

2 Unwell, systemic symptoms, e.g. weight loss

3 Thoracic pain

4 Cancer, steroids, drug abuse, HIV or other significant past history

5 Widespread neurology, e.g. bilateral leg signs

6 Structural deformity

7 Saddle anaesthesia/sphincter disturbance

A full orthopaedic and neurological examination is important. Asymmetry of the iliac crests can be a sign of sacroiliac joint pathology. Scoliosis itself is usually not a cause of pain. Cyanosis, pallor or asymmetry of limb temperature implies vascular or sympathetic involvement. Swelling and loss of hair growth or nail changes support the diagnosis of complex regional pain syndrome (CRPS). Posture gait and station should be examined. Range of motion of the spine does not correlate well with pathology. Testing knee and ankle reflexes in patients with radicular symptoms may determine the level of spinal cord compromise. Weakness with dorsiflexion of the great toe may indicate L5 dysfunction. Lack of plantar flexion of the ankle may indicate S1 root dysfunction. Sensory testing of the medial (L4), dorsal (L5) and lateral (S1) aspects of the foot may also detect nerve root dysfunction. Cervical radiculopathy often affects the C6 roots with sensory loss occurring in the thumb. C7 sensory loss occurs in the middle finger and C8 in the fifth finger. A full understanding of the sensitivity and specificity of the straight leg raising test is needed, in particular the increased specificity and sensitivity of a positive crossed leg raising sign. The femoral stretch test can be considered for upper lumbar root dysfunction [8, 9].

Fibromyalgia syndrome and myofascial pain syndrome are frequent diagnoses in pain clinics. Failure to diagnose muscle pain properly may result in poor treatment outcome, delayed recovery and ineffective, unnecessary surgery. Fibromyalgia syndrome and myofascial pain syndrome both result in sore, stiff, aching, painful muscles and soft tissues. Psychosocial features have been shown to be predictors for developing chronic widespread musculoskeletal pain. Both syndromes share other symptoms including fatigue, poor sleep, depression, headaches and irritable bowel syndrome. Theoretically fibromyalgia should have widespread myofascial trigger points in four body quadrant regions for over 3 months, whereas myofascial pain is thought to be more localized. Aetiology, diagnosis and management of these disorders are a source of controversy [10].

Acute muscle pain is probably universal. It occurs after muscle injury or overuse and resolves after a few days. Chronic muscle pain is extremely common. Most sufferers are able to function satisfactorily in daily activities despite chronic muscle pain. Some report pain-related disability and present a challenge to the healthcare system.

Clinical examination should look for obvious deformity of joints as well as muscular atrophy. If atrophy is suspected, it can be measured. Involved joints should be examined for signs of effusion, instability, and ligament or cartilage pathology. Palpation for areas of spasm or tenderness and for identification of trigger points may be useful in the diagnosis of fibromyalgia. It may be necessary to refer to a rheumatologist if undiagnosed joint problems are found.

Osteoarthritis

Osteoarthritis refers to a clinical syndrome of joint pain accompanied by cartilage loss, hypertrophic bone changes and degeneration. Any synovial joint can develop osteoarthritis but the knees, hips and small hand joints are the common sites affected. Symptoms generally worsen with activity and time and are often insidious in onset. It is important to realize that structural changes commonly occur without accompanying symptoms and radiographic osteoarthritis commonly occurs in the absence of symptoms. Such frequent discordance of osteoarthritis pathology, symptoms and disability means that general assessment features of pain including psychosocial features are important. Joints should be assessed for crepitus and bony changes (e.g. Heberden's nodes) and any signs of inflammation. In advanced disease appropriate discussion with rheumatologists and orthopaedic surgeons is essential.

Neurological assessment

Some brief assessment of mental status is appropriate. Much of the identifiable findings in chronic pain patients will be referable to the peripheral nervous system. Therefore careful evaluation of sensory functions (fine and crude touch, temperature, vibration and position) and motor functions (muscle strength and muscle stretch reflexes) is important. Findings of allodynia, hyperalgesia, dysaesthesia and hyperpathia are useful in cases of suspected neuropathic pain. Signs and symptoms of upper motor neuron dysfunction will provide clues to the existence of potentially painful conditions such as multiple sclerosis or myelopathy due to cervical spinal stenosis. Patients with hemiplegia or hemiparesis may present with central type pain syndromes. It is important to realize that a small fibre peripheral neuropathy may have few clinical signs. Significant new clinical findings may warrant referral to a neurologist.

Functional assessment

Many patients with chronic pain lose the ability to perform activities of daily living. It is important to get an accurate picture of baseline functional ability as a starting point to set therapeutic goals or measure the effectiveness of therapy. Formal questionnaires such as the SF-36 or the sickness impact profile have also been developed [11].

Diagnostic testing

There is no diagnostic test for chronic pain. It is important to remember that finding pathology on diagnostic tests does not necessarily prove that the identified pathology is causing the patient's pain. The sensitivity and specificity of many clinical tests are much lower than we often believe. Nevertheless, diagnostic testing is useful in chronic pain patients for helping to direct treatment and referral.

Plain radiography can sometimes be helpful in musculoskeletal pain to rule out pathology that might require more immediate attention (e.g. an unrecognized fracture or mass lesion). Osteoarthritis presents with loss of joint space, subchondral sclerosis, bone cyst and osteophytes.

Magnetic resonance imaging (MRI) may have a role in back pain, particularly when there is radiculopathy. Disc degeneration, arthritic changes or facet joint degeneration itself is not necessarily painful. The size of a disc protrusion does not correlate with pain level. Most pain physicians like to have this information when evaluating the patient, especially if some intervention is contemplated for the pain. Electromyography (EMG) and nerve conduction studies are of use in patients suspected of having lower motor neuron dysfunction, nerve or nerve root pathology, or myopathy.

In many neuropathic pain syndromes, the results of clinically available laboratory tests are normal. For example, nerve conduction velocity (NCV) and EMG measure only the status of large nerve fibres, and cannot assess small-fibre function. Because many painful neuropathies affect only the small nerve fibres, the NCV and EMG will be normal. Diagnostic testing that could assist in diagnosis (e.g. quantitative sensory testing) often requires specialized equipment and interpretive expertise. Diagnostic imaging is often not useful initially in identifying the anatomical cause of the chronic pain because the abnormalities causing the pain may not be detected. Instead, imaging should be used generally to confirm or rule out the suspected cause of the chronic pain.

Summary

Patient assessment is the start of the therapeutic process. Pain patients are often angry, do not feel that their symptoms are treated seriously and often have a high incidence of coexisting psychopathology, making consultations difficult. While an awkward consultation may be related to unrealistic patient expectations, the clinician should have good interpersonal skills. Adequate consultation time should be given, open-ended questions asked and sympathetic non-verbal skills used. It is often useful to verbalize some of the misconceptions that patients may have, for example 'the doctor thinks my pain is imagined', and an atmosphere of honesty, particularly where diagnostic and therapeutic uncertainty occurs, may help both patient and doctor.

A thorough assessment is essential to the effective management of chronic pain. The patient's history is the most important source of information in assessment. Various assessment questionnaires can be used to complement the history and physical examination. These may give more information about the nature of the pain and other factors known to contribute. Diagnostic tests should be used when appropriate and are mainly used to elucidate aetiological factors.

References

1. Merskey H, Bogduk N (eds). Classification of Chronic Pain: Descriptions of Chronic Pain Syndromes and Definitions of Pain Terms, 2nd edn. IASP Task Force on Taxonomy. Seattle, WA: IASP Press, 1994, 209–14.
2. Waddell G. Volvo award in clinical sciences. A new clinical model for the treatment of low-back pain. Spine 1987; 12:632–44.
3. Macintyre P, Ready LB. Acute Pain Management: A Practical Guide, 2nd edn. London: WB Saunders, 2001.
4. Galer BS, Jensen ME. Development and preliminary validation of a pain measure specific to neuropathic pain: the Neuropathic Pain Scale. Neurology 1997; 48:332–8.
5. Bennett M. The LANSS Pain Scale: the Leeds assessment of neuropathic symptoms and signs. Pain 2001; 92:147–57.
6. Kendall NAS, Linton SJ, Main CJ. Guide to assessing psychosocial yellow flags in acute low back pain: risk factors for long-term disability and work loss. Wellington, NZ: Accident Rehabilitation & Compensation Insurance Corporation of New Zealand, and the National Health Committee, Ministry of Health, 1997.
7. Ewing JA. Detecting alcoholism – the CAGE questionnaire. JAMA 1984; 252:1905–7.
8. Koes BW, van Tulder MW, Thomas S. Diagnosis and treatment of low back pain. BMJ 2006; 332:1430–4
9. Koes BW, van Tulder MW, Peul WC. Diagnosis and treatment of sciatica. BMJ 2007; 334:1313–17.
10. McBeth J, Macfarlane GJ, Benjamin S, Silman AJ. Features of somatization predict the onset of chronic widespread pain. Arthritis Rheum 2001; 44:940–6.
11. Ware JE, Sherbourne CD. The MOS 36-item short-form health survey (SF-36): I. Conceptual framework and item selection. Med Care 1992; 30:473–83.

Further reading

Goucke CR. The management of persistent pain. Med J Aust 2003; 178:444–7.

Chapter 4

Overview of management options

The processing of nociception involves multiple neural pathways, transmitters and receptors. All this suggests that there will never be a single 'magic bullet' analgesic drug. Optimum pain control will therefore require a multimodal approach using several analgesic therapies.

Complete acute pain relief, for example following simple inguinal hernia surgery, is potentially achievable. However, in practice it is not, mainly because patients 'trade off' analgesia against any side-effects experienced from the analgesic therapy and their own expectation that it is normal to 'suffer' some degree of pain following surgery.

Complete analgesia is rarely achievable with chronic pain. Non-malignant nociceptive pain (i.e. mechanical low back pain, osteoarthritis and rheumatoid arthritis) is the most common form of chronic pain. The primary goals here are to improve pain as much as possible, but, most importantly, to optimize physical function and coping with any residual pain.

Integrated care pathways

Pain management techniques fall into four categories: pharmacological, regional analgesia, physical therapy and psychological therapies. Drug therapy has the most research and therefore the largest evidence base behind it. It is possible, for certain conditions, to make specific recommendations for which drug regimens should be used, for example the algorithm for neuropathic pain and the World Health Organization's (WHO) ladder's for cancer pain (*see* Chapter 5). Good practice includes all the therapeutic options, and integrated care pathways (ICPs) are being developed that include all these components.

General principles of drug therapy

In order to choose the most appropriate analgesic medication, a full assessment of the pain problem is required (*see* Chapter 3). The major component of pain needs to be identified as the treatment options are different depending on whether it is nociceptive or neuropathic pain.

A patient should titrate a drug to a suitable dosage and duration until he or she obtains noticeable pain relief or experiences intolerable side-effects. The consensus regarding optimal pharmacological treatment is that the medication should be taken regularly rather than on demand, as it is easier to keep pain at bay rather than trying to control it after it has resurfaced. If there is no relief the drug should be discontinued. If there is partial pain relief, a second drug can be added to the regimen. If patients do obtain benefit, then they can continue on the medication indefinitely, although they should be encouraged to wean off gradually every 6 months or so to ensure that they still require the medication.

The WHO analgesic ladder
The WHO three-step analgesic ladder was developed in the early 1980s as a tool to manage cancer pain (primarily nociceptive in nature). The drugs, which include paracetamol (acetaminophen), non-steroidal anti-inflammatory drugs (NSAIDs), codeine and the stronger opioid drugs, have proved successful in controlling pain in over 80% of patients with cancer (see Figure 4.1).

Paracetamol is well tolerated and seems to be as effective as the NSAIDs in managing the pain of rheumatoid arthritis. There is little effect on the liver at doses of 4 g/day or less. It is indicated for mild-to-moderate pain, but has been shown to reduce the requirements for more potent analgesics in severe acute pain, and cancer pain, and presumably has the same effects with non-cancer chronic pain.

Over two dozen NSAIDs are available. These drugs are useful for musculo-skeletal pain and incident (movement-related) pain. It is logical to try two

Figure 4.1 Drugs used in the World Health Organization's three-step analgesic ladder

Step 1	Paracetamol
	NSAIDs or COX-2 inhibitor
Step 2	Codeine, dihydrocodeine, dextropropoxyphene, meptazinol (often as co-analgesics, i.e. co-codamol)
Step 2→3	Tramadol
Step 3	Morphine, diamorphine, pethidine
	Methadone, fentanyl, buprenorphine
	Oxycodone, hydromorphone

NSAIDs, non-steroidal anti-inflammatory drugs; COX-2, cyclo-oxygenase 2.

or three different NSAIDs in sequence (2–4 weeks each), before judging them to be ineffective. It is well known that patients can obtain benefits or side-effects from one drug and yet not from another in the same family. It is best to start with a drug with the least side-effect profile, and then move on to others if necessary. Consequently most patients will be tried on ibuprofen first, followed by diclofenac or etodolac, for example.

The problem of gastrointestinal (GI) complications led to the development of a new generation of NSAIDs, called COX-2 inhibitors, which block only the cyclo-oxygenase-2 (COX-2) isoenzyme, and therefore have fewer side-effects (e.g. 50% fewer GI complications and no effects on platelet coagulation). They were previously recommended for those patients at risk for peptic ulcer disease, but subsequently were shown to increase the incidence of myocardial infarct and strokes. It transpires now that probably most of the other NSAIDs (except naproxen) suffer from the same problem and we need to evaluate the cardiovascular risk in all patients considered for NSAID therapy [1].

Step 2 and 3 opioids

Use of the less potent Step 2 opioids such as codeine, dihydrocodeine and dextropropoxyphene is commonly but inappropriately practised. These drugs are often not taken on a regular basis and are usually taken combined with paracetamol (500 mg), which limits the daily dose of opioid to eight tablets per day. While the use of compound analgesics may make consumption simpler and compliance better for the patient, it limits optimal opioid titration and is often a more expensive preparation. In addition around 10% of European caucasians are unable to fully metabolize codeine and tramadol, due to pharmacogenetic variances in CYP-2D6. These patients will gain insufficient analgesia from these preparations and will require stronger opioids. It makes sense that, if the decision to use an opioid is made, then a potent Step 3 one should be titrated from a low-dose level up to an appropriate dose to assess response. However, in patients with non-malignant pain, potent Step 3 opioids are rarely used due to concerns, rightly or wrongly, of drug misuse. This situation has recently been improved with the publication of guidelines for opioid use in non-malignant pain [2].

Adjuvant analgesics

Conventional anti-nociceptive analgesics are often ineffective for neuropathic pain. Most of these drugs are called 'adjuvant analgesics' because their primary indication is not for pain (i.e. antidepressants, anticonvulsants and antiarrhythmics). However, many of them are now used more commonly for neuropathic pain than for their approved indication.

Antidepressants and anticonvulsants

The tricyclic antidepressants are the gold standard as they are the most effective and best known. The serotonin selective reuptake inhibitors (SSRIs) are not useful. Amitriptyline is started at a low dose (10–25 mg at night) and gradually increased up to 100 mg if tolerated. Patients must have a full explanation of the rationale for antidepressant therapy, otherwise they may think that the doctor believes their pain to be psychological in origin and may lose trust in them. Similarly, anticonvulsant medication should be started low and titrated slow.

Patients often discontinue the medication because side-effects occur early while onset of analgesia may take several weeks. They must be told to persevere if possible and that they will become tolerant to most of the side-effects after a few days to weeks. One in three patients will get greater than 50% pain relief, regarded as an excellent result for a chronic pain condition (*see* Figure 4.2) [3].

Figure 4.2 The number needed to treat of various adjuvant analgesic drugs for neuropathic pain

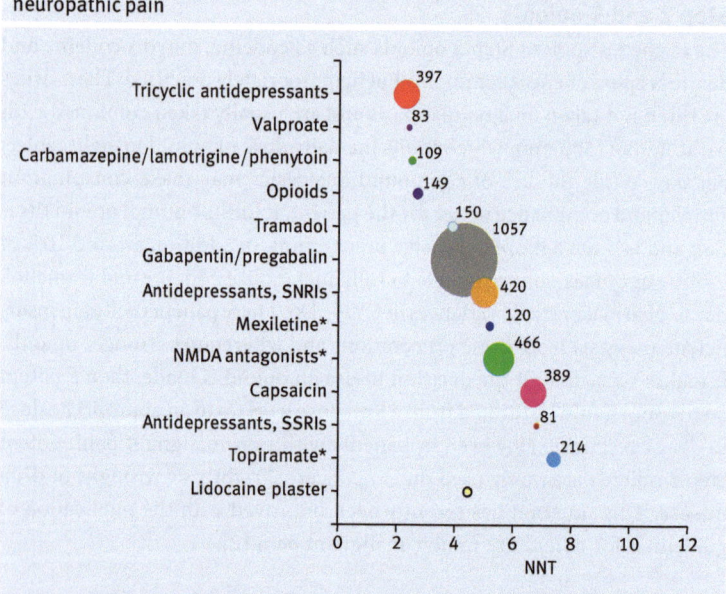

NNT, number needed to treat to achieve pain relief > 50% (i.e. a number of 3 means that three patients will need to be treated for one to obtain the stated objective (usually 50% pain relief)); SNRI, serotonin and noradrenaline reuptake inhibitor; SSRI, selective serotonin reuptake inhibitor.
Reproduced with permission from Finnerup NB, Otto M, McQuay HJ, Jensen TS, Sindrup SH. Algorithm for neuropathic pain treatment: an evidence-based proposal. Pain 2005; 118:289–305.

Figure 4.3 The number needed to treat (NNT) values for 50% pain relief following molar tooth extraction. NSAIDs are superior to opioids for this particular pain model

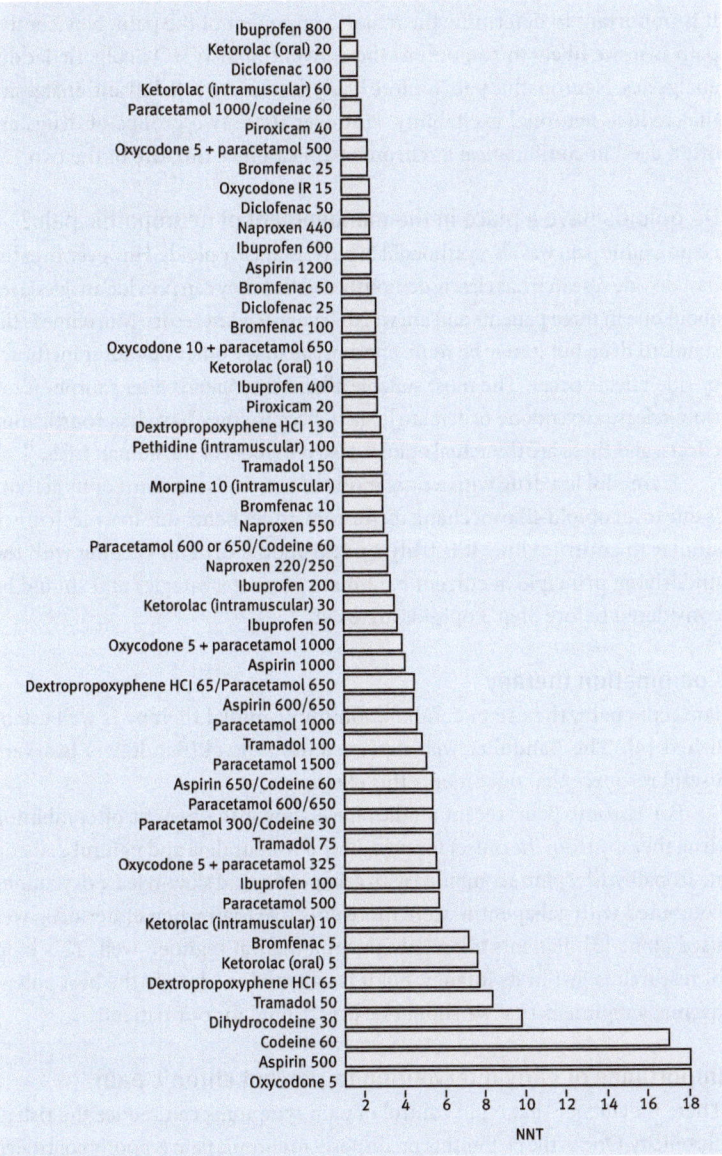

Issues in the pharmacological management of pain

Differentiating neuropathic from nociceptive pain

It is important to determine the major component of the pain. Nociceptive pain is more likely to respond to the conventional WHO analgesic ladder analgesics. Neuropathic pain is more likely to respond to 'adjuvant' analgesics that reduce neuronal excitability. However these two groups of drugs are often used in combination as chronic pain can be a mixture of the two.

Do opioids have a place in the management of neuropathic pain?

Neuropathic pain was always thought to be resistant to opioids. However, over the past decade research has clearly demonstrated that they can provide analgesia for about one in three patients and are worth trying as a last resort. Morphine is the standard drug but it may be more appropriate to try other opioids if inefficacy or side-effects occur. The most suitable alternative opioids after morphine are slow-release oxycodone or fentanyl patch, because they have less constipating effects, and these are the actual opioids tested in most of the human trials.

Tramadol is a drug with a dual mode of activity: one-third of its activity is due to an opioid-like mechanism, the remainder being due to a mechanism similar to amitriptyline. It is truly a multi-modal drug in keeping with the underlying principle of current pain management strategies and should be considered before Step 3 opioids are used.

Combination therapy

For acute pain, the use of combination multi-modal therapy is well established [4]. The Bandolier website (www.jr2.ox.ac.uk/Bandolier) is a very useful resource that documents this clearly.

For chronic pain, recent studies have shown the benefit of combining drug therapy from the outset for post-herpetic neuralgia and painful diabetic neuropathy. Morphine combined with gabapentin, and slow-release oxycodone combined with gabapentin, were more effective than when either drug was used alone [5]. Patients tolerated the combination regimen well. This kind of research is just in its infancy, but it is essential to identify the best polypharmacy regimens that we should be prescribing for our patients.

Importance of early intervention to prevent chronic pain

There is evidence that rapid control of pain symptoms can reduce the risk of chronicity. One of the factors that predisposes to chronic pain is poorly controlled acute pain. While this is not the only factor, it is one of the more readily controlled ones [6]. Aggressive and prompt pain management is practised in order to deliver this goal of reducing the incidence and severity of chronic pain. Designs of research into acute pain have improved over the years but many studies still do not investigate the longer term aspects of recovery (*see* Figure 4.4).

Methods of drug delivery

There are a number of different analgesic drugs available, which can be given by various routes. Concerning opioids in particular, the use of intravenous boluses and patient-controlled analgesia pumps is increasing and has led to an overall improvement in postoperative pain relief (*see* Chapter 5).

Non-pharmacological interventions

This includes other modalities such as interventional regional analgesia, physical therapy rehabilitation, psychological therapies and very occasionally neurosurgery. With the exception of regional analgesia for postoperative pain and psychology-based pain management programmes for chronic pain, the evidence for implementing one specific therapy over another is weak. The exact order of implementation therefore often depends on local availability and experience, side-effect profile, cost and the personal preference of the patient. Often these different therapies are administered simultaneously to provide truly multi-modal analgesia.

Regional analgesia

Regional analgesia describes the local application of drug treatments by regional blockade. Injection of drugs into tissue, for instance into a myofascial 'trigger

---

Figure 4.4 Acute pain outcome parameters. Good acute pain studies must not only document short-term outcomes, but also look at the longer-term recovery profile

↓ Pain VAS – dynamic

↓ Analgesic dose

↓ Side-effects – nausea, vomiting, cardiovascular and respiratory morbidity

↑ Recovery profile:

- i.e. time to oral intake, urine and faecal output, mobility, discharge
- hyperalgesia (alteration in CNS processing) → detected by QST

Health-related quality of life, often regarded as 'soft' outcomes but very relevant

- i.e. global function, patient preferences, cost
- i.e. incidence of chronic pain

QST, quantitative sensory testing; VAS, visual analogue scale.
Data from Wu CL, Raja SN. Optimizing postoperative analgesia: the use of global outcome measures. Anesthesiology 2002; 97: 533–4.

spot' or a perineural injection, means that only a small dose of drug is used and therefore the risk of side-effects is low. Regional analgesia can be applied to any nerve or tissue in the body. This includes somatic nerves (peripheral or cranial), sympathetic nerves and central nerve blocks (epidural and spinals).

For acute pain following surgery, local anaesthetic is used in high concentrations to provide intraoperative regional anaesthesia in addition to postoperative regional analgesia. Epidural and spinal blocks (local anaesthetic often in combination with opioids) are commonly used for abdominal surgery, while peripheral nerve blocks (local anaesthetic alone) are more often used for peripheral limb or body surface surgery (*see* Figure 4.5).

For chronic pain, the indications for performing a nerve block are diagnostic, prognostic or therapeutic. Injections of nerves are first done at a peripheral level for safety reasons, but if unsuccessful can then be performed at progressively more central sites. For inguinal hernia surgery pain, the first procedure might be simple infiltration of scar tissue, followed by lumbar root block, followed by epidural block if required. Blocks often have a beneficial temporary response lasting for days to weeks. The fact that benefits can often outlast the pharmacological activity of the drugs injected is surprising. One possible reason for this is that hyperplasticity is more likely to occur in chronic pain, and blocking the process just for a short while can result in dampening of the neural excitability. The drugs used include a mixture of pharmacological agents. Local anaesthetic drugs are used in a dilute solution in order to block the pain fibres but spare most of

Figure 4.5 Location of possible sites for nerve blockade for acute and chronic pain

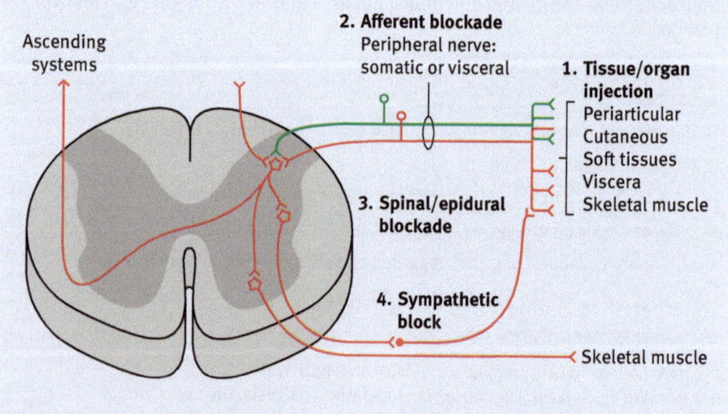

Figure 4.6 The number needed to harm (NNH) of various adjuvant analgesic drugs for neuropathic pain

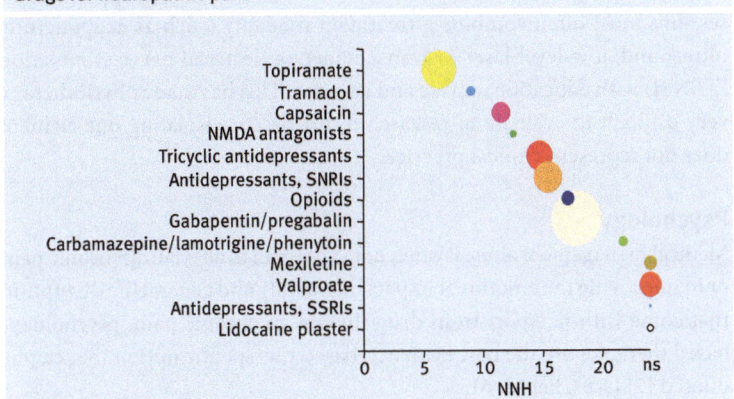

NMDA, *N*-Methyl-D-aspartate; SNRI, serotonin and noradrenaline reuptake inhibitor; SSRI, serotonin selective reuptake inhibitor.
Adapted with permission from Finnerup NB, Otto M, McQuay HJ, Jensen TS, Sindrup SH. Algorithm for neuropathic pain treatment: an evidence-based proposal. Pain 2005; 118:289–305.

the sensory and motor fibres (analgesic rather than an anaesthetic block). Other drugs often injected include opioids, steroids, α_2-agonists (clonidine) and *N*-methyl-D-aspartate (NMDA) antagonists such as ketamine.

Some patients in desperation request a neurolytic block to destroy the nerve permanently. Neurolytic blocks (using alcohol, phenol, cryotherapy or radiofrequency) are rarely performed as the neural system usually regenerates and adapts after 3–6 months. The pain can therefore return or even be worse, and may be accompanied by sensory and motor deficits. These procedures are usually reserved only for the terminally ill patient who will not survive long enough to experience these complications.

Less commonly, a patient will have symptoms that are amenable to more invasive procedures. These include implanted drug delivery systems (epidural and spinals) and dorsal column or intracranial stimulation (*see* Chapter 6). The more invasive treatments should be performed only in appropriately selected patients by centres experienced in such procedures.

Physical therapy

The main aim of physiotherapy in chronic pain is to provide pain relief where possible. It also focuses on the restoration of normal function and helping the patient return to normal physical activities, including going back to employment, through active rehabilitation. Physiotherapy is always delivered as a package; modalities are rarely delivered in isolation. Physiotherapy treatment sessions most often combine a treatment modality (such as acupuncture, ultrasound, low-level laser or transcutaneous electrical nerve stimulation [TENS]) with education, advice and exercise. This has made physiotherapy very difficult to evaluate in research terms because isolating one element does not represent clinical practice.

Psychology

Medical management alone is often not successful in alleviating chronic pain or in improving the emotional impacts, disability and general life disruption that come with it. Apart from drug therapy in chronic pain, psychology-based therapies are the best evidence-based therapeutic option that can be offered [7] (*see* Chapter 6).

Treatment of comorbidities

Chronic pain is a chronic illness and patients often suffer from other medical morbidity. The cause of the pain itself may compromise organ function (i.e. chronic pancreatitis or cancer). Pain itself causes sleep deficits, depression, anxiety, poor appetite and concentration difficulties. Treatment options should not worsen these problems, so the best treatment of comorbidity is to avoid it in the first place by using therapies with the least side-effects. Patients often regard side-effects as more important than efficacy. They are more likely to discontinue a drug if it compromises daily functioning, even if it provides good analgesia.

Special cases

Cancer pain

Patients with cancer often experience more than one pain; one-third will have a single pain, one-third two pains, and one-third three or more pains. The causes of pain include the cancer itself, pain due to treatment (postoperative pain from surgery, radiation therapy and chemotherapy) and coexistent pain such as post-herpetic neuralgia or back pain. Pain management follows the same lines as for non-malignant pain, except that strong opioid drugs are usually started earlier. Multi-modal therapy is usually coordinated by a specialist palliative care team. Anaesthetists or surgeons may be asked for input for specific nerve blocks or neurosurgery (*see* Chapter 6). Pain management incorporates a strong psychological and spiritual component because of the 'end of life' issues. Breakthrough pain is a particularly difficult problem because it is often unexpected and intermittent, usually occurs during movement and is resistant to therapy without causing excessive side-effects during the quiescent times in between breakthrough episodes [8].

Elderly patients

Elderly people generally have a reduced reserve and high incidence of concomitant disease and polypharmacy. Pain assessment can be difficult due to cognitive or communication impairment and altered pain responses. Certain drugs have their limitations. NSAIDs should be used with caution as there is an increased incidence of gastric and renal toxicity. For gastric protection, co-administration of a proton pump inhibitor should be considered. Opioid drugs are effective analgesics but elderly people are more sensitive to sedation and respiratory depression, probably due to altered drug distribution and excretion. Opioid dose titration should be slower and with lower doses. Similarly, with patient-controlled analgesia (PCA), there should be careful titration of the initial dose, avoidance of accumulation by not using background infusions and setting a longer lock-out period. Regional techniques are often better tolerated as they allow a reduction in the use of systemic analgesic drugs.

Children

The assessment of pain in children requires using modified pain scoring systems tailored to their age and understanding. Analgesia should be given by the least painful (and stressful) route and regular assessment of analgesic efficacy is required. Insertion of an intravenous cannula under cover of topical local anaesthetic cream allows painless insertion. Also, rapid control of pain with repeated doses can be given by subcutaneous cannula to avoid repeated intramuscular injection. Children as young as 5 can understand the principles and workings of PCA devices. Psychological support may decrease fear and anxiety of surgical procedures. Drug therapy is the mainstay of postoperative analgesia in children, but the other non-pharmacological methods may also be useful.

References

1. Moskowitz RW, Abramson SB, Berenbaum F, *et al*. Coxibs and NSAIDs – is the air any clearer? Osteoarthritis Cartilage 2007; 15:849–56.
2. Recommendations for the Appropriate Use of Opioids for Non-cancer Pain. London: British Pain Society, 2004 (available from http://www.britishpainsociety.org/book_opioid_main. pdf). Last accessed 8 January 2008.
3. Finnerup NB, Otto M, McQuay HJ, Jensen TS, Sindrup SH. Algorithm for neuropathic pain treatment: an evidence-based proposal. Pain 2005; 118:289–305.

4. Gilron I, Bailey JM, Tu D, et al. Morphine, gabapentin, or their combination for neuropathic pain. N Engl J Med 2005; 352:1324–34.
5. National Health and Medical Research Council. Acute Pain Management: Scientific Evidence, 2nd edn. Canberra: NHMRC, 2005 (available from http://www.nhmrc.gov.au/publications/synopses/_files/cp104.pdf). Last accessed 8 January 2008.
6. Perkins FM, Kehlet H. Chronic pain as an outcome of surgery. A review of predictive factors. Anesthesiology 2000; 93:1123–33.
7. Morley S, Eccleston C, Williams, A. Systematic review and meta-analysis of randomized controlled trials of cognitive behaviour therapy and behaviour therapy for chronic pain in adults, excluding headache. Pain 2000; 80:1–13.
8. Foley KM. Acute and chronic cancer pain syndromes. In: Doyle D, Hanks G, Cherny N, Calman K (eds). Oxford Textbook of Palliative Medicine, 3rd edn. Oxford: Oxford University Press, 2004.

Chapter 5

Pharmacotherapy of pain

Introduction

In order to prescribe for and treat painful conditions pharmacologically it is important to know whether the pain to be treated is nociceptive, neuropathic or mixed in nature. Neuropathic pain in particular may not respond to conventional analgesics. A simple and successful way to use analgesics in most pain conditions requires application of the World Health Organization (WHO) pain ladder [1] and use of multimodal analgesia. This chapter will focus on non-opioid, opioid and anti-neuropathic analgesic medications in current usage and will comment on their efficacy and safe prescription.

The WHO pain ladder was developed to encourage the use of appropriate opioid analgesics in the treatment of cancer pain, but its simple step-wise approach has found utility across all pain conditions. The ladder is shown in Figure 5.1. It starts with simple analgesics such as paracetamol and NSAIDs (non-steroidal anti-inflammatory drugs), then weak opioids and finally strong opioids. Progression up the steps of the ladder, in conjunction with frequent re-assessment of symptoms, provides treatment titrated to the severity of the pain.

The concept of multimodal analgesia involves using smaller doses of many different drugs in an additive or synergistic way to achieve maximum pain relief with fewer side-effects. Thus combining paracetamol and NSAIDs will spare the dose of the weak or strong opioid used when progressing to the next rung of the ladder.

Regular prescribing of analgesics maintains the plasma concentration at a therapeutic level, thereby reducing breakthrough pain. In general all chronic pain conditions should employ this fixed daily dosing of longer-acting preparations, to provide steady analgesia and permit daily functioning. However, all conditions (particularly acute and cancer pain) need as-required prescriptions of fast-acting analgesics to treat incident pain or exacerbations of pain.

Figure 5.1 The WHO analgesic pain ladder

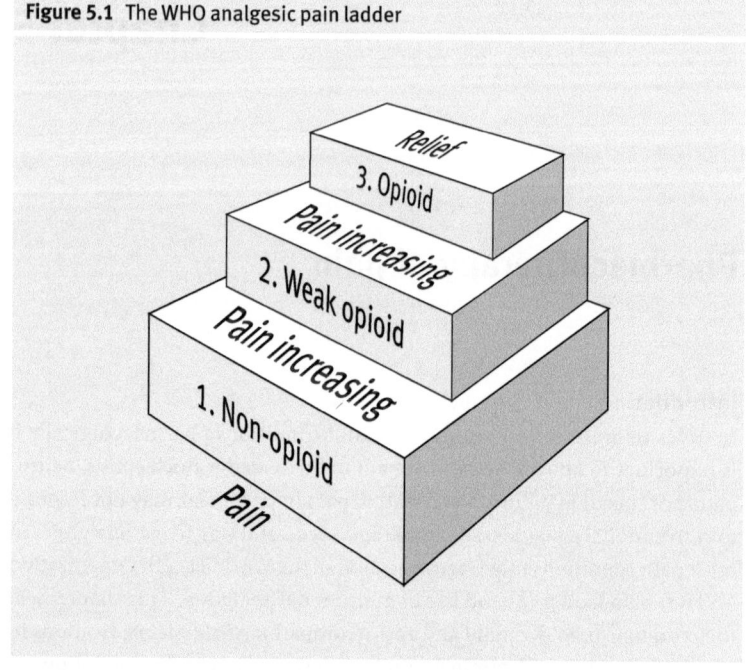

Adapted with permission from World Health Organization. Cancer Pain Relief and Palliative Care (Technical Report Series 804). Geneva: WHO: 1990: 1–75.

While most analgesics can safely be prescribed in combination with other analgesics it is important to be aware of important relative and absolute contraindications, particularly when dealing with NSAIDs and anti-neuropathic medications that affect serotonin metabolism. An understanding of the pharmacokinetics of these drugs will permit their safe use and avoid drug interactions when dealing with patients with hepatic or renal disease.

Non-opioid analgesics

This category of analgesics encompasses paracetamol (acetaminophen), phenazone and NSAIDs. The last group can be further subdivided according to affinity for the cyclo-oxygenase (COX) enzyme isotypes. Newer anti-inflammatories in this group target the COX-2 enzyme (COX inhibitors – COXIBs). Figure 5.2 lists the NNTs of these analgesics (number of patients needed to have treatment for one patient to achieve a specific outcome, e.g. usually 50% pain relief) [2].

Figure 5.2 NNT of non-opioid analgesics in acute pain

Drug	Dose (mg)	NNT
Paracetamol	1000	3.8
Phenazone	1000	1.9
Diclofenac	50	2.3
Ibuprofen	200	2.7

NNT, number needed to treat.
NNT for 50% pain relief, based on data from Moore A, Edwards J, Barden J, McQuay H. Bandolier's Little Book of Pain. Oxford: Oxford University Press, 2003; and Schug SA, Manopas A. Update on the role of non-opioids for postoperative pain treatment. Best Pract Res Clin Anaesthesiol 2007; 21:15–30.

Paracetamol

Paracetamol is an analgesic and antipyretic medication. Its mode of action is still uncertain but it is thought to act centrally near the hypothalamus and possibly through a COX-3 mechanism. It may also have an action on serotoninergic systems and a peripheral action on bradykinin-sensitive chemoreceptors.

Presented as oral, intravenous or rectal preparations, paracetamol can be readily administered to fasting patients perioperatively. Its oral bioavailability is almost 90%, but rectal absorption is variable and unreliable. Oral and intravenous doses of 15 mg/kg, up to a maximum of 4 g/day, can be safely administered in adults, although the total dose should be reduced appropriately in children and low-weight adults as excessive doses can cause hepatotoxicity.

While the majority of paracetamol is metabolized in the liver safely through glucuronidation, a small proportion is metabolized via a separate cytochrome P450 system that can lead to the generation of oxygen free radicals when glutathione stores are exhausted. This causes local tissue necrosis and, if severe, can lead to hepatic failure and death. Caution should be exercised when using paracetamol in patients with hepatic impairment or when alcohol and other hepatic enzyme-inducing drugs have been used.

The evidence for using paracetamol in chronic conditions has been looked at mainly in osteoarthritis groups. In these studies paracetamol has performed well against placebo and, although its benefit may not be as great as that of the NSAIDs, its safety profile is very good and this makes it the first-line analgesic for all pain states. It can spare the dose of opioid drugs by around 20% [3–5].

A promising future development for paracetamol is in combination with nitric oxide (NO) as nitroparacetamol (or nitroacetaminophen) [6]. This experimental formulation has been studied in rats and found to be up to 20 times as potent as paracetamol alone. Interestingly the compound does not display the cardiovascular or hepatotoxic side-effects seen with paracetamol. It is thought that its augmented effects and anti-inflammatory actions occur from the slow release of NO. Further studies using sub-therapeutic doses in combination with fentanyl highlight a potent opioid-sparing effect and the possibility of reduced opioid-induced hyperalgesia [7]. If this work can be replicated in human trials then nitroparacetamol may have an important role in the future of pain management.

Phenazone (antipyrine)

This analgesic also has antipyretic and anti-inflammatory properties. It is thought to act via a COX-3 mechanism in the dorsal horn of the spinal cord. Given in a dose of 500 mg to 1 g orally, it has been studied in many pain conditions including migraine. Although it has a similar efficacy to paracetamol it has a far poorer safety profile and can cause agranulocytosis, anaphylaxis, haemolysis and nephrotoxicity. This extensive side-effect profile means that phenazone is rarely used as an oral analgesic and its use is restricted in many countries [8].

NSAIDs

This class of painkiller also has antipyretic and anti-inflammatory actions. The name was derived to make a distinction from the corticosteroid class of drugs that also reduce inflammation. Figure 5.3 lists some of the common NSAIDs.

NSAIDs such as ibuprofen, diclofenac and naproxen act on the COX-1 and COX-2 enzymes to reduce the synthesis of inflammatory mediators. The COX enzyme mediates the breakdown of arachidonic acid into prostaglandins and

Figure 5.3 NSAIDs and COXIBs

Drug	Dose in chronic use (mg per 24 h)	Gastrointestinal risk
Ibuprofen	2400	Low
Diclofenac	150	Intermediate
Naproxen	1000	Intermediate
Celecoxib	400	Low
Etoricoxib	60	Low
Lumaricoxib	100	Low

COXIB, cyclo-oxygenase-2 inhibitor; NSAID, non-steroidal anti-inflammatory drug.

thromboxanes. The latter has an effect on endothelial function and clotting, the former has complex proinflammatory actions and essential homoeostatic functions. Most of the analgesia and anti-inflammatory effect comes from prostaglandin reduction, but the non-specific nature of the blockade causes many of the side-effects seen with NSAIDs and was the stimulus for the development of COX-specific drugs (COXIBs) such as celecoxib, etoricoxib and lumiracoxib. A separate enzyme, lipoxygenase, breaks arachidonic acid into leukotrienes, which can also mediate inflammation peripherally, but most NSAIDs do not interfere with this pathway. Figure 5.4 illustrates the pathway from tissue injury to inflammation.

The NSAIDs are particularly useful for musculoskeletal pain and dental pain and are used perioperatively to spare opioid dosing by around 30–40% [9, 10]. Compared with paracetamol, NSAIDs are superior in postoperative pain from dental surgery, but have comparable efficacy following orthopaedic surgery. There is not enough evidence to make any conclusion with major abdominal, minor gynaecological or ENT surgery [5].

As there is no difference in efficacy between selective and non-selective anti-inflammatory drugs their prescription should be based on safety and cost. The UK Committee for Safety in Medicines (CSM) currently advises that if used they should be prescribed at the lowest effective dose for the shortest period of time. This advice is due to the common and serious side-effects that

Figure 5.4 Role of cyclo-oxygenase

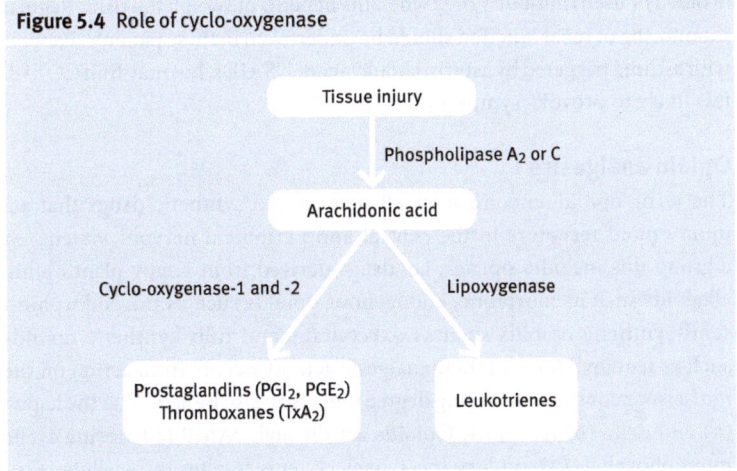

As well as being proinflammatory mediators following tissue injury, prostaglandins (PGI_2 and PGE_2) and thromboxanes (TxA_2) have important physiological functions in the gastrointestinal tract, renal tract and vasculature. See text for details.

occur with NSAIDs through prostaglandin inhibition. These include gastric ulceration, hypertension, sodium and water retention leading to peripheral oedema and congestive heart failure, non-union of bone, renal impairment, thrombotic cardiac events and bronchoconstriction triggering asthma. All anti-inflammatories affecting COX can increase the risk of myocardial infarction (MI) and thrombotic stroke, but the COX-2-selective drugs are particularly dangerous in this regard and should be avoided in patients with cardiovascular disease. Although from meta-analysis the number needed to harm (NNH) for MI has been quoted at 333 [11], the event is serious and may occur in the short term. The COX-2-selective drugs are advantageous over conventional NSAIDs when the risk of GI side-effects and bleeding is increased (e.g. in patients with previous or current peptic ulcer disease or who are on drugs predisposing to peptic ulcers and in post-trauma or perioperative bleeding situations). GI side-effects, including gastric and duodenal ulceration and bleeding, are common and can occur with short courses of only 5–7 days. There is a 2–4% incidence of ulceration in NSAID users, three to four times the rate in the general population. The use of COX-2 anti-inflammatories reduces the occurrence of GI complications [4, 9, 11, 12] and the addition of an antacid or proton pump inhibitor (PPI) can further reduce gastric erosion. However, up to 40% of bleeds occur in the lower GI tract.

In elderly people or those with renal impairment, NSAIDs should be avoided or used cautiously only when the benefits outweigh the risks. Regular monitoring of renal function should be undertaken in these patients. Patients with asthma triggered by aspirin should avoid NSAIDs, but may find COXIBs less likely to provoke symptoms [10].

Opioid analgesics

The term 'opioid' encompasses all natural and synthetic drugs that act upon opioid receptors in the central and peripheral nervous system. As a group this includes opiates, i.e. drugs derived from poppy plant opium alkaloids such as morphine, endogenous opioids such as the endorphins, semi-synthetic opioids such as oxycodone, and fully synthetic opioids such as fentanyl. Most of their analgesic activity occurs from action on the mu (μ) receptor but to a varying degree there may also be action on the kappa (κ) and delta (δ) receptors. Opioids act through cAMP (adenosine cyclic monophosphate) secondary messenger systems to alter intracellular Ca^{2+} concentrations and hyperpolarize neuronal cell membranes, thereby decreasing synaptic responses in the pain pathways. Although they are primarily used to augment the intrinsic endorphin analgesia pathways, they also impact on the mesolimbic dopaminergic reward pathways and can lead to dependence states in susceptible individuals.

Unfortunately the concepts of tolerance, dependence and addiction are frequently confused and have led to a reluctance to prescribe morphine and related analgesics. It is not uncommon for patients using opioids to be stigmatized and treated with suspicion, particularly when requesting additional analgesia.

Tolerance, which is not a phenomenon isolated to opioids, describes the situation where an increasing dose of drug is required to achieve the same clinical benefit. In the case of opioids, this diminution of effect over time occurs due to uncoupling of the intracellular pathways or activation of anti-analgesic pathways via NMDA (N-methyl-D-aspartate) mechanisms [13]. Ultimately, as the dose increases to maintain analgesia, there are often significant side-effects, which may necessitate opioid rotation.

Dependence has distinct physical and psychological components which, when not described fully, can lead to the mislabelling of patients as dependent in an 'abusive' connotation. With chronic use every patient will develop physical dependence to opioids due to physiological adaptation; long-term exposure to opioids alters intercellular processes to a new set point that will be destabilized by the abrupt cessation of treatment. This is classically manifest as autonomic hyper-reactivity with CNS and cardiovascular system lability causing symptoms such as arousal, sleeplessness, irritability, psychomotor agitation, piloerection, tachycardia and hypertension. Reintroduction of the medication will abort the physical withdrawal symptoms, but, if the drug is not reinstated, over time the symptoms will settle as the body re-establishes a new equilibrium without the drug. Psychological dependence occurs in susceptible individuals, through genetic predisposition and learned reinforcement. Typically, dysphoria and craving sensations develop when the drug is removed. A formal diagnosis of substance dependence under psychiatric classification [14] requires more than three criteria from those listed in Figure 5.5.

Addiction describes a maladaptive state of misuse that impacts negatively on work, home or school functioning, and is manifest as compulsive use or continued abuse despite harm and craving. For a long time it was believed that only a very small percentage of patients became addicted to analgesic medication, but in the last 20 years rates of between 3% and 50% have been quoted, depending on the criteria used [15]. Of these studies, one using DSM-IV criteria quoted an incidence of substance dependence in sickle cell disease patients at around 30%, but when opioid-seeking behaviour for analgesia was excluded from the data the incidence fell to less than 5%. The

Figure 5.5 DSM-IV criteria for substance dependence

Diagnosis requires three or more from:

1	Tolerance
2	Withdrawal
3	Increased dosing or duration of use
4	Unsuccessful weaning attempts
5	Increased time spent obtaining drug
6	Loss of social or recreational activities through drug use
7	Continuation of use, despite knowledge of physical or psychological harm

Based on criteria from APA: Diagnostic and Statistical Manual of Mental Disorders, 4th edn. Washington, DC: American Psychiatric Association (APA), 1994.

occurrence of dependence and addiction phenomena is therefore higher than was previously believed in chronic pain conditions, but is still not a problem for the vast majority of patients. There are complex genetic, biochemical and social triggers as well as personality traits that facilitate addiction. Although no screening tools are particularly robust at detecting individuals prior to initiating medication, avoidance or caution when using opioids is advised in those patients who display risk-taking behaviour or poor impulse control, or have a personal or family history of addiction. Patients who appear overly attentive to their medication at clinic assessment, who complete prescriptions too early, request replacement prescriptions or obtain opioids from more than one source should be screened for substance dependence or addiction risk before treatment is continued.

The prescription of an opioid is appropriate for moderate-to-severe pain conditions but patients should be warned about the potential side-effects, particularly when long-term use is planned. Almost a quarter of patients discontinue opioid therapy due to intolerable side-effects [16]. Most frequently these include constipation, nausea, drowsiness (particularly when initiating treatment and with subsequent dose increases), pruritus and respiratory depression. With prolonged treatment opioids can also cause immunosuppression, via stimulation of the hypothalamic–pituitary–adrenal axis that impairs lymphocyte function. Chronic use also suppresses gonadotrophins and testosterone production leading to sexual dysfunction and mood imbalance. A rare but recognized side-effect is opioid-induced hyperalgesia where, paradoxically, increasing the dose of the opioid exacerbates pain. This occurs through phosphorylation of the opioid pathways secondary to increased protein kinase C expression. This happens when NMDA, chole-cystokinin (CCK), dynorphin and glial cells interact in complex pain conditions [17]. Opioid-induced hyperplasia should be suspected if the quality of the pain changes and becomes more diffuse and widespread with a temporal relationship to dose increases. Efforts should be made when commencing opioid therapy to reduce the common side-effects by co-prescribing laxatives and antiemetics and optimizing polypharmacy to avoid concomitant CNS depressants. If myoclonus or delirium develops, then assessment for dehydration, systemic infection or drug interaction should be initiated, as these are common precipitants. If conservative management fails then dose reduction or opioid rotation may alleviate the symptoms.

Clinically, opioids may be subdivided into weak and strong subclasses and used as progressive steps on the pain ladder. Codeine, dihydrocodeine, dextropropoxyphene and tramadol are weak opioids whereas morphine, oxycodone, methadone, hydromorphone, fentanyl and buprenorphine are strong opioids. Clinically relevant prescribing points for these drugs will be outlined in the following sections, but more comprehensive pharmacokinetic data can be found in clinical pharmacology textbooks [18].

Weak opioids

Codeine
This opiate has around a tenth of the potency of morphine and good oral bioavailability. Codeine has a maximum daily dose of 240 mg and dosing should be reduced in patients with renal failure. Around 10% of codeine is converted to morphine in the body, providing much of its analgesia. It is used in oral and intramuscular preparations and is most commonly prescribed in combination with paracetamol for mild-to-moderate pain (co-codamol). Codeine undergoes hepatic metabolism by the cytochrome P450 enzyme CYP-2D6, which displays genetic variability, such that 10% of the European population are either 'ultrafast metabolizers' or 'slow metabolizers'. This results in some patients gaining fast and potent analgesia and others who claim no benefit from codeine. Constipation is a common side-effect.

Dihydrocodeine
This opioid was developed as an antitussive and is one-and-a-half times more potent than codeine. It can be used to increase analgesia in patients who gain benefit from codeine. It is prescribed up to 240 mg/day in divided doses of 30–60 mg. It has an oral bioavailability of 20% and is frequently prescribed in combination with paracetamol for moderate pain (co-dydramol). It undergoes hepatic metabolism and has some very potent active metabolites, such as dihydromorphine glucuronide. Constipation is a common side-effect.

Dextropropoxyphene

This weak opioid has now been discontinued in the UK due to its side-effect profile. It is still available in the USA, Australia and Scandinavia. Used for mild-to-moderate pain in combination with paracetamol (co-proxamol), the metabolites of dextropropoxyphene also have some local anaesthetic action. However, its abuse potential (euphoria) and its side-effects of heart failure (cardiac conduction abnormalities including QT widening), respiratory failure (in combination with alcohol and CNS depressants) and mood alteration (suicide), have led to restriction on its use by the CSM. Patients using combination analgesics that contain dextropropoxyphene should be switched to a safer codeine formulation.

Tramadol

This synthetic opioid has dual action, being both a μ agonist and a serotonin (5-HT) reuptake inhibitor. The latter action facilitates descending inhibitory pathways to reduce pain afferent input. Tramadol has high oral bioavailability and can be used up to a maximum of 400 mg/day in divided doses as immediate or slow-release formulations. It has oral and intravenous (IV) preparations and is metabolized in the liver to produce one active metabolite. Its dose should be reduced in renal failure and care should be exercised when using tramadol in patients on tricyclic antidepressants (TCAs), monoamine oxidase inhibitors (MAOIs) or serotonin selective reuptake inhibitors (SSRIs) because serotonin syndrome can occur. This syndrome results from a build-up of 5-HT due to the synergistic effects of the aforementioned drug classes, and can cause CNS and cardiovascular system instability and in some cases death. Although rare, if the combined prescription of these drugs is warranted on clinical grounds, patients should be advised of symptoms and signs to watch out for. These include irritability or altered conscious level, sweating, GI upset, flushing and pyrexia. Symptoms generally occur within 48 hours of commencing treatment, but can be delayed and occur in patients who have been on long-term therapy. Treatment is supportive, with removal of one or all of the drugs. Tramadol causes less constipation than other opioids. It has been used in patient-controlled analgesia (PCA) techniques with a bolus dose of 10–20 mg and a lock-out of 6–10 minutes.

Strong opioids

Morphine

This is the most common opiate used in the UK. It can be used orally, intravenously, intramuscularly or subcutaneously, although its oral bioavailability is only 50%. A conversion of 1:3 should be employed when converting between oral and intravenous preparations. The intravenous dose is 0.1 mg/kg in divided doses. The onset of action of morphine is around 6 minutes and the duration of action is approximately 96 minutes (the period at which the concentration is above 80% of maximum) and so it should be titrated gradually to effect [19]. Morphine causes histamine release that can transiently drop the blood pressure, particularly when given as a bolus. It is metabolized in the liver to morphine-3-glucuronide (M3G) and morphine-6-glucuronide (M6G), which are secreted via the kidney. M6G has analgesic effects but due to its water-soluble nature has a slow effect–site equilibration across the blood–brain barrier and can take up to 7 hours to reach steady state. Some of the side-effects of morphine, in particular those of tolerance and hyperalgesia, have been attributed to the build-up of M3G, but evidence for this is conflicting. The dose of morphine should be reduced in patients with renal impairment.

Morphine is frequently used postoperatively in PCA techniques. Typically it is given as a 1-mg bolus with the lock-out set to 5 minutes. This offers the best balance between analgesia and safety [20]. There is a 1% incidence of respiratory depression with PCA use and this risk is increased when background infusions are used [21]. In general, the use of a background infusion should be avoided in opioid-naïve individuals; however, an infusion can be used safely to replace the morphine equivalent of slow-release oral preparations in patients who are fasting. Appropriate monitoring and management protocols should be in place to detect and treat serious side-effects. Figure 5.6 shows a typical PCA device and Figure 5.7 outlines the treatment algorithm for common PCA side-effects.

While there is no difference in outcome or length of hospital stay with PCA versus conventional morphine analgesia (intramuscular, subcutaneous), patients prefer the control that they have with PCA and gain better analgesia [22]. The incidence of severe pain occurring during different postoperative analgesic techniques has been quoted at 10.4% for PCA versus 29% for intramuscular morphine, and where possible PCA morphine should be utilized over intramuscular or subcutaneous therapies to improve analgesia [23].

Efforts should be made when ceasing PCA to gradually wean opioid usage to prevent sudden withdrawal. By calculating the previous 24-hour requirement of intravenous morphine, an oral 12-hour sustained-release morphine dose can be calculated by multiplying by a factor of 1.5, or an oral 12-hour slow-release oxycodone dose can be calculated by taking the IV morphine dose directly. For example, if 20mg of IV morphine was used in the preceding 24 hours then the patient should commence on sustained-release morphine

Figure 5.6 PCA (patient-controlled analgesia) device

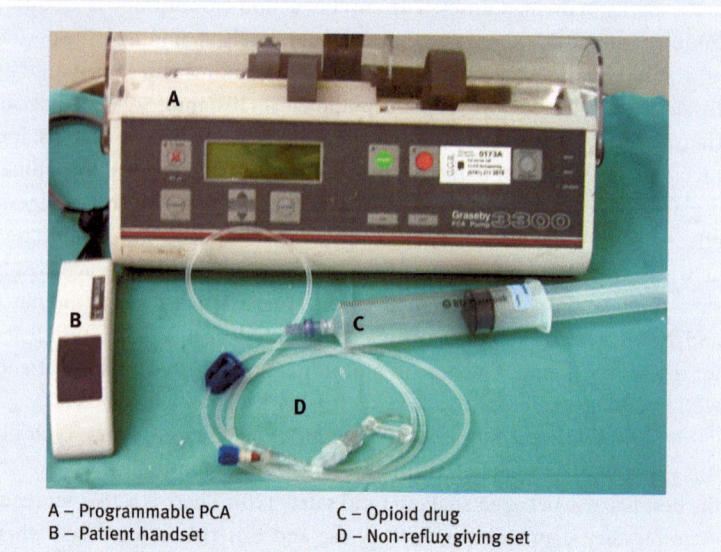

A – Programmable PCA
B – Patient handset
C – Opioid drug
D – Non-reflux giving set

A typical PCA device has adjustable bolus dose, lock-out time and background infusion parameters. The opioid is locked within the pump and is used with a non-reflux giving set system.

30mg twice daily or slow-release oxycodone 20mg twice daily when the PCA stops. Alternatively, multiplying the IV morphine dose by a factor of three gives the oral equianalgesic dose and this facilitates appropriate dosing when rotating from morphine to any other opioid.

Hydromorphone

This drug is similar in action and metabolism to morphine, but is between five and ten times more potent. It comes in intravenous and oral preparations, including sustained-release formulations, although its oral bioavailability is only 35%. It is more soluble than morphine, which offers advantages when used in intrathecal pumps and low-volume delivery systems. Its dose should be reduced in renal impairment. It can be used in a PCA delivery system with a bolus dose of 0.2–0.4 mg and a lock-out of 6–10 minutes.

Oxycodone

This μ agonist opioid has a high oral bioavailability of almost 90%, which facilitates oral dosing of immediate-release or sustained-release prepara-

Figure 5.7 PCA set up, trouble-shooting, and side effects

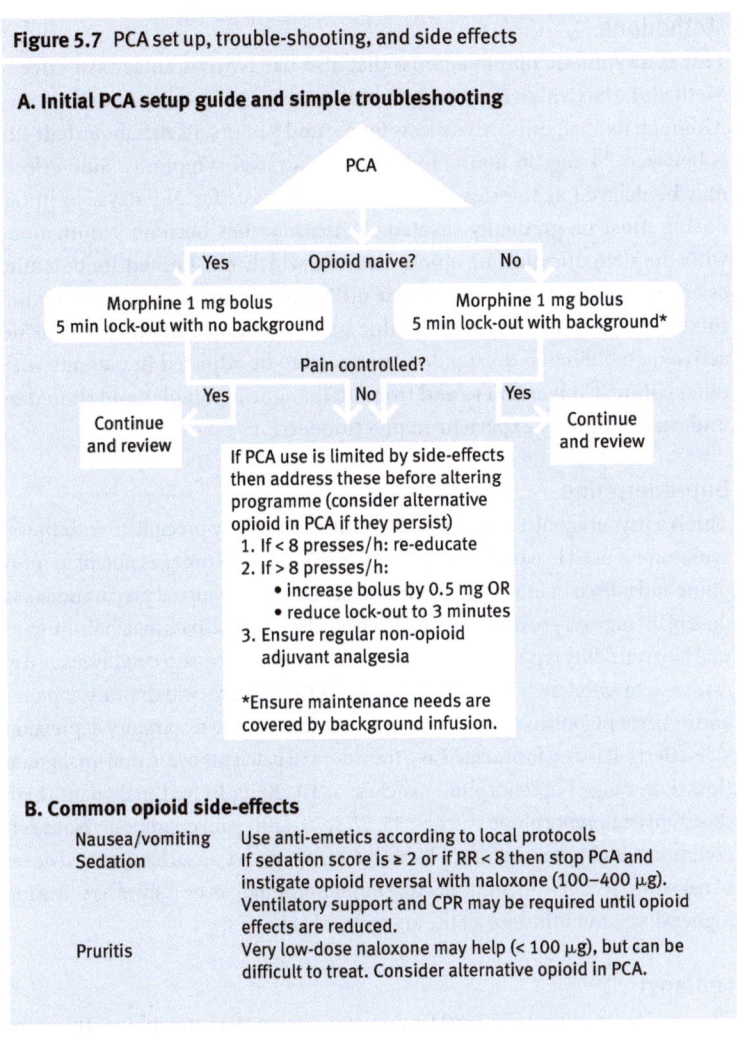

A. Initial PCA setup guide and simple troubleshooting

PCA

Opioid naive?

Yes — Morphine 1 mg bolus 5 min lock-out with no background

No — Morphine 1 mg bolus 5 min lock-out with background*

Pain controlled?

Yes — Continue and review

Yes — Continue and review

No —
If PCA use is limited by side-effects then address these before altering programme (consider alternative opioid in PCA if they persist)
1. If < 8 presses/h: re-educate
2. If > 8 presses/h:
   • increase bolus by 0.5 mg OR
   • reduce lock-out to 3 minutes
3. Ensure regular non-opioid adjuvant analgesia

*Ensure maintenance needs are covered by background infusion.

B. Common opioid side-effects

Nausea/vomiting	Use anti-emetics according to local protocols
Sedation	If sedation score is ≥ 2 or if RR < 8 then stop PCA and instigate opioid reversal with naloxone (100–400 μg). Ventilatory support and CPR may be required until opioid effects are reduced.
Pruritis	Very low-dose naloxone may help (< 100 μg), but can be difficult to treat. Consider alternative opioid in PCA.

CPR, cardiopulmonary resuscitation; PCA, patient-controlled analgesia; RR, respiratory rate.

tions. It is slightly more potent than morphine and causes less histamine release. Intravenous preparations have a faster onset and are twice as potent as oral formulations. Although some accumulation of metabolites occurs in patients with renal impairment, this has not been associated with clinical effects and immediate-release formulations of oxycodone have been used safely in this patient group.

Methadone

This is a synthetic opioid agonist that also has NMDA antagonist effects. Methadone has a high oral bioavailability and comes in syrup or tablet form. Although its analgesic activity lasts for around 8 hours, its metabolic half-life is between 24 and 36 hours, reducing withdrawal symptoms. Side-effects may be delayed as the steady state does not occur for 3–5 days, so initial dosing must be gradually titrated. Methadone has become synonymous with the detoxification of opioid addicts, which has limited its potential as an analgesic, but it has particular utility in pain management for opioid rotations and in treating neuropathic pain conditions. Methadone has no active metabolites so dosing does not need to be adjusted in patients with renal failure. Conversion to and from methadone is complex and should be undertaken only by experienced practitioners.

Buprenorphine

This is a partial agonist at the opioid receptor and so may precipitate withdrawal symptoms if used in a patient already on opioids. It is 25 times as potent as morphine and is used in intravenous, intramuscular and sublingual preparations at a dose of 0.3 mg every 6–8 hours. It undergoes extensive first-pass metabolism, so its oral bioavailability is poor. It is used in moderate-to-severe pain conditions and to assist opioid withdrawal therapies. Its longer half-life reduces withdrawal symptoms and its partial agonism results in a ceiling on euphoria and respiratory depression side-effects. It is also formulated as a transdermal patch for use in non-malignant (low dose range buprenorphine patches; 5, 10, 20 µg/h) and malignant (high dose range buprenorphine patches; 35, 52.5, 70 µg/h) pain conditions. Nausea is common with buprenorphine. (Although resistant to reversal by standard doses of naloxone, recent work indicates that buprenorphine can be fully reversed using higher doses and infusions of the antagonist [24].)

Fentanyl

This synthetic opioid is 50–80 times more potent than morphine. It is used perioperatively in a dose of 1 µg/kg with an onset of action of 5 minutes and has a duration of action of around 30 minutes. It is fat soluble and used commonly to augment anaesthetic neuroaxial blockade in combination with local anaesthetics. Its fast onset and potency make it an attractive option to treat incident and breakthrough pain, and it has been developed as lozenges and sublingual sprays for this effect, as its oral bioavailability is poor at 33%. It has a pulmonary bioavailability of 67% via modern aerosol technologies [25] and this may prove to be a useful delivery modality for cancer pain treatment. In chronic painful conditions and particularly cancer pain, fentanyl patches are available in doses of 12.5–100 µg/h. The patches must be changed every 72 hours, and the slow onset and offset and depot nature of this formulation make it unsuitable for acute pain management.

Fentanyl can be used safely in PCA techniques at a dose of 20–40 µg bolus with a lock-out of 5–10 minutes. It is particularly useful in patients with renal impairment where the build-up of morphine metabolites can cause significant side-effects.

A fentanyl iontophoretic transdermal system (ITS) has recently been developed [26, 27]. This battery-operated, needle-free device gives a bolus of 40 µg fentanyl with a 10-minute lock-out. It can administer up to 80 doses and last for up to 24 hours. It has similar patient satisfaction scores and efficacy as conventional PCA techniques. Its advantages include increased patient mobility, a reduction in infection risk as there is no skin puncture and less nursing input with a reduction in programming errors. It is an expensive single-use modality, but when the logistics and costing of large-scale PCA devices and maintenance are taken into account, the cost of the ITS system is significantly improved. Limitations include its fixed dosing programme. It can also cause local skin reactions and the electronics within the device can fail. At the moment it is licensed only for in-hospital use, but the potential for day-surgery use is obvious.

Opioid selection and recommendations for chronic pain

All opioids can reduce painful symptoms by around 30%, as demonstrated by short-term trial work [28]. As there is insufficient evidence to support one opioid over another, selection should be based on the nature of the pain and guided by patient tolerability, with therapy titrated to analgesia and functional improvement goals. Agonists of the µ receptor are useful in nociceptive pain; tramadol and methadone have theoretical benefit in neuropathic pain states due to their additional mechanisms of action, though this has not yet been demonstrated clinically. If pain is poorly controlled despite escalating doses of opioid, or if side-effects are intolerable, then opioid rotation should be considered. Most of the evidence for this procedure is taken from work in cancer pain and more than 50% of patients benefit from switching [29]. It is safer to dose on the low end of the conversion as differing receptor affinities and narrow therapeutic ranges may result in significant clinical changes. The use of a more frequent short-acting breakthrough medication will be required during the transition period, typically equivalent to one-sixth of the total daily dose. Figure 5.8 lists the approximate equi-analgesic doses of some common opioids. It should be noted that these ratios are not reciprocal and clinicians should be guided by patient response, especially when titrating to and from methadone [29,30].

Figure 5.8 Equi-analgesic doses

In acute pain 10 mg morphine (p.o.) is equal to:		In chronic or cancer pain To rotate opioid from morphine (p.o.), divide dose by:	
Oxycodone	5 mg	÷ 5	= Hydromorphone
Methadone	5 mg	÷ 1.5	= Oxycodone
Codeine	100 mg	÷ 100	= Fentanyl
Tramadol	50 mg	÷ 4–12*	= Methadone
Hydromorphone	2.5 mg		
Buprenorphine	0.2 mg s.l.		

Patches and approximate 24-hour morphine equivalents or PCA replacements†

Fentanyl 25 μg/h	= 60–90 mg morphine/24 hours (~ 1.25 mg/h)
Buprenorphine 5 μg/h	= 5–10 mg morphine/24 hours (~ 0.06–0.13 mg/h)
Buprenorphine 35 μg/h	= 30–60 mg morphine/24 hours (~ 0.5–1.0 mg/h)

Due to physiological and pharmacological variability between patients and drugs, patient response should be monitored during rotation and dose conversion should be rounded down initially, with more frequent breakthrough analgesia, until a new stable dose is established. Conversions are between oral doses unless otherwise stated.
*Conversion from morphine to methadone is non-linear. As a guide if the 24-hour morphine dose is < 100 mg, divide by 4, between 100 mg and 300 mg, divide by 8 and for dose conversion from > 300 mg morphine divide by a factor of 12. There may be delayed sedation side-effects from methadone, due to slow drug equilibration. Dose adjustment should occur after 72 hours.
†Due to the slow onset (6–12 hours) and offset of transdermal analgesics (the drug reservoir prolongs the half-life to 18 hours for fentanyl and > 24 hours for buprenorphine) care should be taken to ensure that there is not an opioid overdose, when converting from patches, and that there is sufficient analgesia prescribed until the patch commences, when converting to transdermal therapy.
PCA, patient-controlled analgesia; p.o., per os; s.l., sublingual
Based on data from Mercadante S, Bruera E. Opioid switching: A systematic and critical review. Cancer Treat Rev 2006; 32:304–15; and McIntyre P, Ready BL. Acute Pain Management: A Practical Guide, 2nd edn. Oxford: Elsevier, 2002.

Current recommendations for the use of opioids in non-malignant pain [31] include open discussion of the benefits and side-effects of treatment with a focus on specific goals and outcomes, including functional gains and pain score improvements. The idea of a 'contract' with the patient is gaining ground whereby failure to achieve benefit from the opioids will result in their cessation and the patient has an obligation to submit to toxicology monitoring and attend regular follow-up. Opioids should be used in conjunction with multidisciplinary care in chronic pain management and as an adjunct to non-opioid analgesics in acute and cancer pain therapy.

Analgesics for neuropathic pain

Non-opioid and opioid analgesics have a role to play in dampening pain transmission in the final common pathways within the CNS in neuropathic pain states. However, using drugs that specifically target the sodium, calcium and NMDA receptors, which are altered when nerves are injured, offers far more powerful analgesic routes in these patients. Drugs that are effective in neuropathic pain come from the antidepressant, anticonvulsant, local anaesthetic or NMDA antagonist families. The efficacy of these drugs has been collated to form NNT tables for differing types of neuropathic pain in an attempt to facilitate prescribing [32,33]. Figure 5.9 lists some NNTs for common antineuropathic agents. This information allows extension of the pain ladder when dealing with neuropathic pain. As a guide, the first step is commonly antidepressants, followed by anticonvulsants, then local anaesthetic agents and finally NMDA antagonists (Figure 5.10).

Antidepressants

These include TCAs, SSRIs and serotonin and noradrenaline (norepinephrine) reuptake inhibitors (SNRIs) [34].

Figure 5.9 NNTs for antineuropathic agents

Drug	NNT
TCA	3.1
SSRIs	6.8
SNRIs	5.5
Gabapentin	4.7
Pregabalin	4.7
Carbamazepine	2.0
Valproate	2.8
Ketamine	7.6
Lidocaine	4.4

NNT, number needed to treat; SNRI, serotonin and noradrenaline (norepinephrine) reuptake inhibitor; SSRI, serotonin reuptake inhibitor; TCA, tricyclic antidepressant.
NNT is the number of patients treated for one patient to achieve more than 50% pain relief.
Based on data from Sindrup SH, Jensen TS. Efficacy of pharmacological treatments of neuropathic pain: an update and effect related to mechanism of drug action. Pain 1999; 83:389–400; and Attal N, Cruccu G, Haanpaa M, et al. EFNS guidelines on pharmacological treatment of neuropathic pain. Eur J Neurol 2006; 13:1153–69 for pooled neuropathic conditions.

Figure 5.10 Neuropathic pain ladder

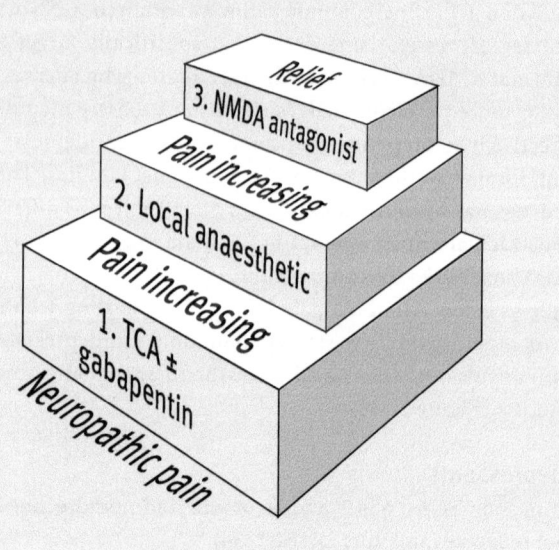

Based on World Health Organization. Cancer Pain Relief and Palliative Care
(Technical Report Series 804). Geneva: WHO, 1990: 1–75.
NMDA, N-methyl-D-aspartate; TCA, triglyceride antidepressant.

TCAs

These are the most efficacious drugs for most neuropathic pain conditions
and are used first line. They act via histaminic, muscarinic and serotoninergic
receptors both centrally and peripherally. They are used in lower doses than
are therapeutic for depression and their utility is limited by side-effects, of
which dry mouth, sedation and urinary retention are the most common,
but cardiovascular changes including arrhythmia can occur. As the TCAs
are dangerous in overdose, they should be avoided in patients with suicide
risk or poor impulse control. Increasingly TCAs are being used for acute
and perioperative neuropathic pain conditions [35,36]. Early use of these
drugs may limit the progression and severity of chronic pain development,
but dosing and duration of treatment remain uncertain. Amitriptyline,
as either 10 mg or 25 mg once daily at night, is the most common way to
initiate treatment. If sedation is a problem with this then imipramine or
nortriptyline may be tried instead. Although some patients describe benefit
after a day or two, it usually takes up to 2 weeks for the majority of patients
to notice any pain relief.

SSRIs/SNRIs

These drugs are less effective than the TCAs, but have a far better safety profile. They act to augment descending inhibitory pathways by reducing reuptake of serotonin and/or noradrenaline. They are useful in patients who cannot tolerate TCAs or when mood disturbance (depression) is to be treated simultaneously [37]. Duloxetine has been studied in painful diabetic peripheral neuropathy with success [38] and venlafaxine, an SNRI, has shown benefit in chronic polyneuropathies. Otherwise, as a class they have an NNT around 6 and should be trialled according to tolerability. Their onset of action is slow and it may take 14–28 days for benefit to become apparent. Side-effects include GI upset and weight gain.

Anticonvulsants

These agents act on sodium and calcium channels to dampen excitability within the nervous system. The doses used are less than those required to control epilepsy and are titrated to effect. As a class the anticonvulsants have an NNT of around 5 and there is little evidence to support one over another except on side-effect profile [39]. The most commonly used include gabapentin, pregabalin, sodium valproate, carbamazepine and lamotrigine. Common side-effects are GI upset, sedation and weight gain.

Gabapentin

This acts on $\alpha_2\delta$ Ca^{2+} channels, which are up-regulated after nerve injury. Gabapentin has the most benign side-effect profile of all the anti-convulsants and does not require monitoring during use, so it tends to be the first choice. Initiated at 100–300 mg, it can be titrated to a maximum of 1.8 g/day in three divided doses. Gabapentin has been trialled perioperatively with promising effects on acute pain management [40,41].

Pregabalin

This is a newer drug, similar in action and efficacy to gabapentin. With similar side-effects but linear pharmacokinetics it can be titrated more accurately, with twice-daily dosing of between 75 mg and 300 mg.

Carbamazepine

This has been used to treat trigeminal neuralgia, but is less well tolerated than the newer anticonvulsants and requires haematological monitoring for liver toxicity and bone marrow depression. Blood dyscrasias, skin rashes and cerebellar side-effects are common. It is commenced at 100 mg twice daily.

Sodium valproate

This is generally well tolerated, but can cause hepatic dysfunction and GI upset, so liver function tests (LFTs) should be monitored. Transient hair loss can also occur. It is titrated from 100 mg twice a day.

Lamotrigine

Less frequently used due to the need for haematological monitoring (thrombocytopenia) and potential severe skin reactions (Steven–Johnson syndrome). Therapy can be initiated at 25 mg once daily for 2 weeks, and increased gradually by 25 mg each week to effect. The usual dose is around 50–200 mg/day.

Local anaesthetics

In nerve injury the sodium channel populations expressed on the nerves are altered. The up-regulated Na^+ voltage-gated channels (Na_v) are particularly sensitive to blockade by local anaesthetic (LA) agents, but systemic toxicity, especially cardiovascular and CNS side-effects, restrict the utility of this therapy. To avoid these effects but still provide benefit, LAs such as lidocaine tend to be used in discrete nerve blocks, as brief intravenous infusion techniques, as oral equivalents (mexiletine) or topically in patch formulations. A Cochrane review of the efficacy of LAs in placebo-controlled trials was favourable; their benefit is similar to that gained from other antineuropathic agents [42]. The transdermal 5% lidocaine patch is useful in elderly and frail patients with post-herpetic neuralgia, or isolated scar pain, as systemic effects are negligible [43]. Mexiletine is an oral analogue of lidocaine, but tolerability is poor due to nausea and diarrhoea, so very few patients gain long-term benefit from its use. LA blocks of peripheral or central nervous structures can provide a depot of agent near the damaged nerve and temporarily block afferent conduction.

NMDA antagonists

Ketamine, an anaesthetic agent, is the most commonly used NMDA antagonist. The NMDA receptor is an important contributor to the wind-up mechanism and perpetuation of neuropathic pain. Blockade of this receptor can reverse intracellular mechanisms that contribute to opioid tolerance and central sensitization. At subanaesthetic doses, ketamine has preventive effects on pain when used in the acute setting [44,45]. Side-effects limit its utility, in particular hallucinations and nightmares, although the use of benzodiazepines can reduce these. Most frequently ketamine is used perioperatively in a single dose (0.4 mg/kg) around the time of surgery, in patients at high risk of developing chronic pain, or for those with poorly controlled acute pain. It can be given as an infusion postoperatively, intravenously or subcutaneously at a dose of 0.1 mg/kg/h, in patients with morphine tolerance or to regain pain relief in cancer patients whose pain has decompensated. Anecdotally, some patients gain long-term pain relief from brief infusions of ketamine. This is thought to occur due to NMDA closure breaking the sensitization cycle in the dorsal horn, but there is as yet no way to predict who will benefit from its use and many patients fail to tolerate even small doses [46].

Other drugs used to treat neuropathic pain include cannabinoid derivatives and capsaicin cream. The former are limited by side-effects and the latter, although efficacious with an NNT of 6, may be poorly tolerated due to skin irritation in up to 10% of patients.

Special groups

Pregnancy/lactation
Up-to-date information can be found in medicine prescribing formularies (e.g. *British National Formulary*) and practitioners should consult the formulary before prescribing unfamiliar medications. With the exception of paracetamol all analgesics should be avoided if possible during pregnancy. Opioids, but not tramadol, can be used, but there is a risk of withdrawal syndrome and respiratory depression in the neonate. For antidepressants and anticonvulsants, if the benefits outweigh the risks then they can continue to be prescribed. Typically this guidance refers to the risk of suicide and status epilepticus and not pain relief. NSAIDs should be avoided as they can close the ductus arteriosus and cause pulmonary hypertension in the newborn.

While the concentration of drugs in breast milk is generally too low to cause harm, most manufacturers recommend avoidance unless clinical need is apparent. In this situation it is important to discuss with the mother whether breast milk expression or feeding with formula milk should take place. Paracetamol, opioids and LAs can all be used safely.

Elderly people
With increasing age, pain thresholds increase but pain tolerance reduces. Arthritis and other degenerative conditions are common and require regular analgesia. Deteriorating renal function and hepatic metabolism affect drug clearance and polypharmacy, and comorbidities increase the likelihood of drug interaction. Elderly patients are more likely to be affected adversely by the sedating side-effects of analgesics. Communication difficulties and

memory impairment may worsen compliance and pain expression. However, despite these changes pain can be treated successfully and safely in this population [47].

Through slow titration of analgesics and use of the pain ladder, appropriate drugs can be administered safely ('start low, go slow'). Pharmacy dosette boxes can aid compliance by separating analgesics into 'times' and 'days'. If long-acting medications are to be used then patients should be monitored for longer at the commencement of therapy and at dose changes, as equilibration may be delayed due to poor renal clearance and so CNS depressant effects may not manifest for 2–3 days. Co-prescribing of laxatives and anti-emetics should occur when using opioids and short-acting analgesics for breakthrough pain should be routinely available.

Summary

By using multimodal analgesia principles and following either the nociceptive or neuropathic pain ladders, almost all pain conditions can be successfully controlled pharmacologically. The earlier use of anti-neuropathic medication will reduce the severity and progression to chronic pain.

Awareness of the absolute and relative contraindications of the most common analgesics and cautious prescribing in the special groups outlined above will reduce drug interactions and promote safety.

References

1. World Health Organization. Cancer Pain Relief and Palliative Care (Technical Report Series 804). Geneva: WHO, 1990: 1–75.
2. Moore A, Edwards J, Barden J, McQuay H. Bandolier's Little Book of Pain. Oxford: Oxford University Press, 2003.
3. Nikles CJ, Yelland M, Del Mar C, Wilkinson D. The role of paracetamol in chronic pain: an evidence-based approach. Am J Ther 2005; 12:80–91.
4. Schug SA, Manopas A. Update on the role of non-opioids for postoperative pain treatment. Best Pract Res Clin Anaesthesiol 2007; 21:15–30.
5. Hyllested M, Jones S, Pedersen JL, Kehlet H. Comparative effect of paracetamol, NSAIDs or their combination in postoperative pain management: a qualitative review. Br J Anaesth 2002; 88:199–214.
6. Moore PK, Marshall M. Nitric oxide releasing acetaminophen (nitroacetaminophen). Dig Liver Dis 2003; 35:S49–60.
7. Gaita'n G, Ahuir FJ, Herrero JF. Enhancement of fentanyl antinociception by subeffective doses of nitroparacetamol (NCX-701) in acute nociception and in carrageenan-induced monoarthritis. Life Sci 2005; 77:85–95.
8. Aronson JK (ed.). Phenazone. In: Meyler's Side Effects of Drugs: The International Encyclopedia of Adverse Drug Reactions and Interactions. Oxford: Elsevier, 2006: 2794.
9. Buvanendran A, Reuben SS, Kroin JS. Recent advances in nonopioid analgesics for acute pain management. Tech Reg Anaesth Pain Manag 2007; 11:19–26.
10. Langford RM, Mehta V. Selective cyclo-oxygenase inhibition: its role in pain and anaesthesia. Biomed Pharmacother 2006; 60:323–8.

11. Moskowitz RW, Abramson SB, Berenbaum F, *et al.* Coxibs and NSAIDs – is the air any clearer? Osteoarthritis Cartilage 2007; 15:849–56.
12. Lyseng-Williamson KA, Curran MP. Lumiracoxib. Drugs 2004; 64:2237–46.
13. Watkins L, Hutchison MR, Ledeboer A, *et al.* Glia as the 'bad guys': Implications for improving pain control and the clinical utility of opioids. Brain, Behav Immun 2007; 21:131–46.
14. APA: Diagnostic and Statistical Manual of Mental Disorders, 4th edn. Washington, DC: American Psychiatric Association, 1994.
15. Ballantyne JC, LaForge KS. Opioid dependence and addiction during opioid treatment of chronic pain. Pain 2007; 129:235–55.
16. McNicol E. Opioid Side-Effects. Pain: Clinical Updates, Volume XV; Issue 2. Seattle, WA: International Association for the Study of Pain 2007 (available online from http://www.iasp-pain.org).
17. Koppert W. Opioid induced hyperalgesia – pathophysiology and clinical relevance. Acute Pain 2007; 9:21–34.
18. Sasada M, Smith S. Drugs in Anaesthesia and Intensive Care, 3rd edn. Oxford: Oxford University Press, 2003.
19. Grass J. Patient controlled analgesia. Anesth Analg 2005; 101:S44–61.
20. Owen H, Plummer JL, Armstrong I, *et al.* Variables of patient controlled analgesia 1: Bolus size. Anaesthesia 1989; 44:7–10.
21. MacIntyre P. Safety and efficacy of patient controlled analgesia. Br J Anaesth 2001; 87:36–46.
22. Hudcova J, McNicol E, Quah C, Lau J, *et al.* Patient controlled opioid analgesia versus conventional analgesia for postoperative pain. Cochrane Database of Systematic Reviews 2006 (4): CD003348.
23. Lehmann K. Recent developments in patient controlled analgesia. J Pain Symptom Manage 2005; 29:S72–89.
24. Dahan A. Opioid induced respiratory failure: new data on buprenorphine. Pall Med 2006; 20:3–8.
25. Farr SJ, Otulana BA. Pulmonary delivery of opioids as pain therapeutics. Adv Drug Deliv Rev 2006; 58:1076–88.
26. Langford RM, Rawal N. A new needle free PCA system. The fentanyl iontophoretic transdermal system. Acute Pain 2006; 8:151–3.
27. Minkowitz HS. The fentanyl iontophoretic transdermal system: a review. Tech Reg Anesth Pain Manage 2007; 11:3–8.
28. Kalso E, Edwards JE, Moore RA, McQuay HJ. Opioids in chronic non-cancer pain: a systematic review of efficacy and safety. Pain 2004; 112:372–80.
29. Mercadante S, Bruera E. Opioid switching: A systematic and critical review. Cancer Treat Rev 2006; 32:304–15.
30. McIntyre P, Ready BL. Acute Pain Management: A Practical Guide, 2nd edn. Oxford: Elsevier, 2002.
31. Recommendations for the Appropriate Use of Opioids for Persistent Non-Cancer Pain. London: British Pain Society, 2004 (available from http://www.britishpainsociety.org/opioid_doc_2004.pdf). Last accessed 27 January 2008.
32. Sindrup SH, Jensen TS. Efficacy of pharmacological treatments of neuropathic pain: an update and effect related to mechanism of drug action. Pain 1999; 83:389–400.
33. Attal N, Cruccu G, Haanpaa M, *et al.* EFNS guidelines on pharmacological treatment of neuropathic pain. Eur J Neurol 2006; 13:1153–69.
34. Saarto T, Wiffen PJ. Antidepressants for neuropathic pain. Cochrane Database of Systematic Reviews 2005 (3): CD005454.
35. Bousher D. The effects of pre-emptive treatment of post-herpetic neuralgia with amitriptyline: a randomised, double-blind, placebo controlled trial. J Pain Symptom Manage 1997; 13:327–31.

36. Kalso E, Tasmuth T, Neuvonen PJ. Amitriptyline effectively reduces neuropathic pain following treatment of breast cancer. Pain 1996; 6:17–24.
37. Finnerup NB, Otto M, McQuay HJ, Jensen TS, Sindrup SH. Algorithm for neuropathic pain treatment: An evidence based proposal. Pain 2005; 118:289–305.
38. Wernicke JF, Pritchett YL, D'Souza DN, et al. A randomised controlled trial of duloxetine in diabetic peripheral neuropathy. Neurology 2006; 67:1411–20.
39. Wiffen P, Collins S, McQuay H, et al. Anticonvulsant drugs for acute and chronic pain (review). Cochrane Database of Systematic Reviews 2005 (3); CD001133.
40. Seib RK, Paul JE. Pre-operative gabapentin for postoperative analgesia: A meta-analysis. Can J Anaesth 2006; 53:461–9.
41. Hurley RW, Cohen SP, Williams KA, et al. The analgesic effects of perioperative gabapentin on postoperative pain: A meta-analysis. Reg Anesth Pain Med 2006; 31:237–47.
42. Challapalli V, Tremont-Lukats IW, McNicol ED, Carr DB. Systemic administration of local anaesthetic agents to relieve neuropathic pain. Cochrane Database of Systematic Reviews 2005 (4): CD003345.
43. Galer BS, Jensen MP, Ma T, et al. The lidocaine patch 5% effectively treats all neuropathic qualities: results of a randomised, double-blind, vehicle controlled, 3 week efficacy study with the use of the neuropathic pain scale. Clin J Pain 2002; 5:297–301.
44. Katz J, McCartney CL. Current status of pre-emptive analgesia. Curr Opin Anaesth 2002; 15:435–41.
45. Bell RF, Dahl JB, Moore RA, Kalso E. Perioperative ketamine for acute neuropathic pain. Cochrane Database of Systematic Reviews 2006 (1): CD004603.
46. Hocking G, Visser EJ, Schug S, Cousins MJ. Ketamine: Does life begin at forty? Pain: Clinical Updates (Volume XV; Issue 3. Seattle, WA: International Association for the Study of Pain 2007 (available online from http://www.iasp-pain.org).
47. Auburn F, Marmion F. The elderly patient and postoperative pain treatment. Best Pract Res Clin Anaesthesiol 2007; 21:109–27.

Chapter 6

Non-pharmacological management of pain

Interventional and neurosurgical approaches

Introduction

Interventional pain procedures have their own place in the treatment algorithm of resistant chronic pains. The advantages of these techniques are that they are usually a one-off treatment over a period of months and do not require maintenance therapy and, if effective, patient compliance is good.

Because of the potential complications of interventional procedures, they are usually performed after a failed trial of non-invasive therapies. No single specific intervention totally relieves persistent pain; they should be considered only as one therapeutic option among the overall treatment plan.

In chronic pain, the goals of the interventional treatment include decreasing the frequency and/or the intensity of the pain, improving the patient's functional capacity, and enhancing the patient's ability to cope with the residual pain.

Classification

Invasive procedures include nerve blocks, injections, ablative procedures, implants, and neuromodulation. A classification of these is given in Figure 6.1.

Nerve blocks

Nerve blocks in pain management are used for both diagnostic and therapeutic purposes. Generally, diagnostic nerve blocks are carried out for the following reasons:

- To evaluate and compare the roles of the sympathetic and somatosensory nerves in maintaining the pain.
- To identify the particular nerves that convey the pain, or to alter neuromuscular function.

Figure 6.1 A classification of invasive approaches to pain management

Blocks: procedures designed to temporarily interrupt the nervous system activity, usually with local anaesthetics. They can be:

- neuroaxial (epidural, selective nerve root blocks)
- peripheral nerves (intercostal, suprascapular, ilio-inguinal, upper and lower extremity blocks)
- autonomic: stellate ganglion, lumbar sympathetic chain

Injections: joint injections, trigger point injections

Counterstimulation: acupuncture, physical therapy and transcutaneous nerve stimulation

Neuromodulation techniques:

- spinal cord stimulation
- peripheral nerve stimulation
- intrathecal drug delivery

Neuroablative procedures: invasive procedures that permanently interrupt nervous system activity:

- chemical: alcohol, phenol
- physical: burning by radiofrequency denervation, freezing by cryoneurolysis
- surgical

Diagnostic blocks can help clarify the cause of pain. For example, low back pain can result from many causes – the paravertebral muscles, intervertebral discs, surrounding ligaments, vertebral bodies or facet joints. If the back pain is relieved by facet joint denervation, it supports the diagnosis of facet joint pathology as the cause. Similarly, leg pain relieved by sympathetic denervation implies that the main component of pain is conveyed by sympathetic rather than somatic nerve fibres.

In performing a diagnostic block for sympathetic pain, the clinician must choose a site at which the anaesthetic is unlikely to affect somatic nerves, as this would interfere with interpretation. Similarly with somatic pain, a very small amount of local anaesthetic is injected at the specific nerves. Fluoroscopy or ultrasound can be used to locate the injection site precisely.

For a diagnostic block, 0.5% bupivacaine with or without steroids is used. Steroids currently used are depot preparations of methylprednisolone and triamcinolone. The doses generally range between 40 and 80 mg for epidural injection and between 20 and 40 mg for selective nerve root block.

Common diagnostic/therapeutic blocks

Epidural steroid injections

Radicular pain is a sharp, shooting pain in the distribution of a spinal nerve (usually to the arm or leg in the case of cervical or lumbosacral radiculopathy). This type of pain occurs due to nerve root irritation by inflammatory mediators extruded from an intervertebral disc or actual compression caused by a disc, spinal stenosis or spondylolisthesis. Injection of steroid around nerve roots can be effective for the treatment of radicular pain [1]. Steroids reduce the inflammation and swelling around the nerve root. Once this result is achieved, resumption of normal activity and participation in focused physical therapy and rehabilitation can be expected.

Epidural injections are performed if pain is bilateral and involves multiple level nerve roots. These injections can be performed at different levels (caudal, lumbar, thoracic or cervical region) depending on the site of pain. An expert performs these blocks in a sterile setting (day-case surgery theatre) to minimize the risk of infection. The benefit of an epidural injection can vary from 1 week to 6 months.

Selective nerve root blocks

These are performed if only one or two nerve roots are involved in ongoing radicular pain. The block is done using radiological guidance and local anaesthetic/steroid injection is deposited at the target nerve root. At times this block is performed as a diagnostic procedure on request by a surgeon. If the patient gets pain relief for an appropriate time after the injection, this will support an indication for discectomy or decompression of the nerve root for long-term pain relief.

Peripheral nerve blocks

These blocks are performed if pain is in the distribution of peripheral nerves (Figure 6.2). They are performed using local anaesthetics with or without steroid.

Autonomic ganglion blocks

Sympathetic nerve blocks are performed for diagnostic or therapeutic purposes.

There are a number of chronic pain conditions in which the sympathetic nervous system is involved in ongoing pain generation. Examples

Figure 6.2 Peripheral nerve blocks

Nerve blocked	Pain problem
Ilio-inguinal nerve	Post-hernia pain
Occipital nerve block	Occipital neuralgia
Intercostal nerve block	Chest wall pain after thoracotomy
Suprascapular nerve block	Shoulder pain

of this are complex regional pain syndrome, post-amputation pain and ischaemic leg pain. Sympathetic ganglia such as the stellate ganglion, coeliac plexus, lumbar sympathetic chain and superior hypogastric plexus (*see* Figure 6.3) are blocked using local anaesthetic (with or without steroid), physical heat-mediated damage (radiofrequency lesioning) or neurolytic solutions. Another way of blocking the sympathetic supply to part of a limb is by performing an intravenous regional block using a ganglion blocker, e.g. guanethidine.

Injections

Joint pain is a common cause of pain, especially in elderly people. The affected joints are injected using local anaesthetics and steroids. Depo-steroids are added to prolong the duration of relief.

Sacroiliac joint pain frequently contributes to low back pain. The patient usually has tenderness over the sacroiliac joint. This joint is blocked under radiological guidance using local anaesthetic and steroid injections.

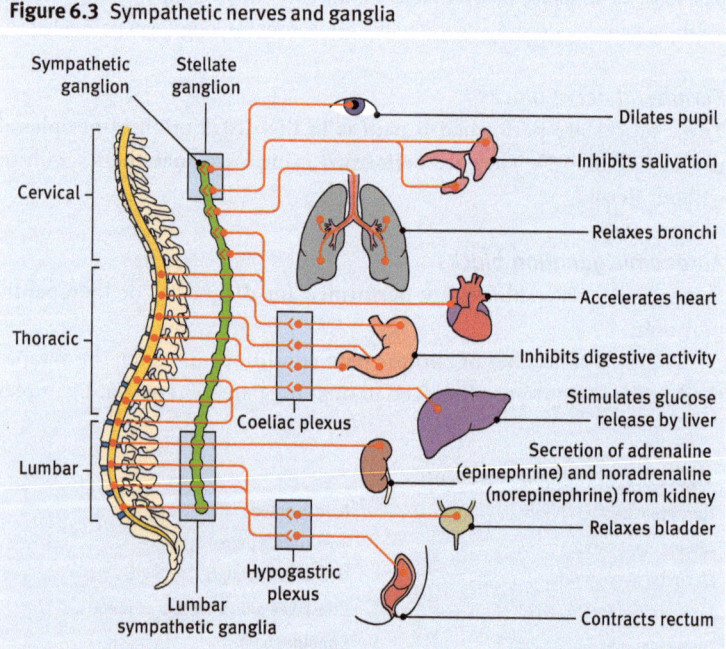

Figure 6.3 Sympathetic nerves and ganglia

Sympathetic ganglion

Stellate ganglion

Dilates pupil

Inhibits salivation

Cervical

Relaxes bronchi

Accelerates heart

Thoracic

Inhibits digestive activity

Stimulates glucose release by liver

Coeliac plexus

Secretion of adrenaline (epinephrine) and noradrenaline (norepinephrine) from kidney

Lumbar

Relaxes bladder

Hypogastric plexus

Lumbar sympathetic ganglia

Contracts rectum

Facet joint injection

The facet joint (also known as the zygapophyseal joint) is the joint between the articular processes of adjacent vertebrae. Lower back pain or neck pain can result from facet joint degenerative arthropathy related to old age or trauma. Facet joint pain causes non-radicular low back pain or neck pain, which worsens with extension and lateral bending of the spine.

Facet joint injections are performed under fluoroscopic guidance. This block can be performed as a diagnostic procedure to clarify the cause of pain or as a therapeutic option in order to provide respite. If the patient's pain is relieved after facet joint injection, then joint denervation is performed to prolong the duration of pain relief. The facet joint is denervated by radiofrequency lesioning of the joint nerves (the medial branch of the posterior primary ramus of a spinal nerve).

Trigger point injections

The trigger point is a band of muscle spasm that on palpation triggers pain. Trigger points are commonly present in a patient with myofascial pain syndrome, which is characterized by spontaneous and evoked pain in the muscles. Needling or injection of trigger points is performed for diagnostic or therapeutic purposes and to facilitate the physical therapy. The reproduction of pain during injection into the muscle and subsequent pain relief is the hallmark of trigger point pain. Trigger points are usually injected with local anaesthetics, sometimes botulinum toxin and rarely steroids.

Counterstimulation

Acupuncture

Acupuncture has been used as a therapy for a variety of illnesses for more than 3,000 years. According to classical Chinese teaching, energy (qi) flows through a number of channels (meridians) in the body (see Figure 6.4). Imbalance in the flow of energy in different parts of the body leads to disease and pain. The meridians can be influenced by needling of acupuncture points to unblock obstruction and/or allow excess energy to be dissipated and thus corrects imbalance in the flow of energy. It has been estimated that there are approximately 360 classic acupuncture points in the human body.

The exact mechanism of action remains unclear but the most widely accepted acupuncture model proposes that needling of tissue sends impulses to the spinal cord and activates three centres – the spinal cord, midbrain, and hypothalamus–pituitary system. This activation leads to the release of neurotransmitters (e.g. endogenous opioids) and hormones.

Figure 6.4 An example of meridians used in acupuncture

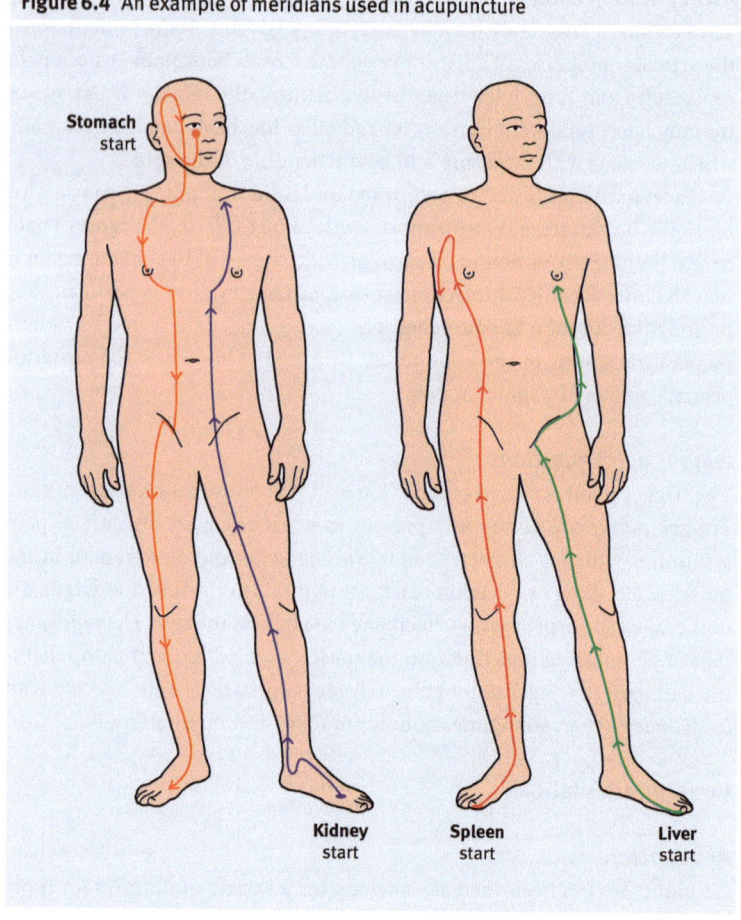

Acupuncture is safe, cost-effective, and devoid of any major side-effects or complications. It is effective in some patients with myofascial pain, fibromyalgia, low back pain, osteoarthritis and headache. Short-term benefit is the limitation.

Physical therapy

Physical therapy aims to improve or restore the function and therefore prevent disability. In chronic pain, treatments that focus solely on elimination of pain will very likely fail to alter the illness and disability behaviour of the chronic pain patient. The treatment should address function in addition to pain, to promote more independence and a level of tolerance. Physical therapy interventions include:

- Education and self-management: explaining to patients their diagnosis and pathology is helpful in reducing fear and eliminating catastrophizing. When patients understand their pathology and agree with goals of interventions, they are more likely to be compliant with the intervention offered.
- Active modalities: stretching exercise, strengthening exercise and endurance exercise.
- Counterstimulation techniques: electrical stimulation, ultrasound, heat, and cold are commonly used in physical therapy.

Transcutaneous electrical nerve stimulation

TENS is the application of current through electrodes placed on the skin (*see* Figure 6.5). This activates large-diameter (Aβ) fibres. There are two main stimulation patterns: low-frequency (1–4 Hz), high-intensity, long pulse-width signals that cause visible muscle contractions, and a high-frequency (50–100 Hz), low-intensity signal that causes a tingling or buzzing sensation. A small portable device with two or four leads is used to produce the low-voltage electrical current.

TENS works on the principles of the gate control theory of pain modulation. High-frequency stimulation 'closes the gate' for pain signals at spinal cord level by stimulation of Aβ-fibres, whereas low-frequency stimulation is thought to activate the pain-inhibiting descending pathways.

Figure 6.5 Transcutaneous electrical nerve stimulation

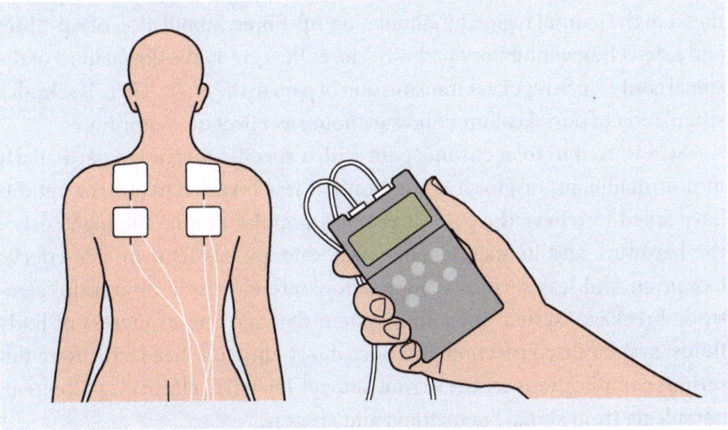

TENS is used to treat low back pain, refractory angina pain and osteoarthritis pain.

There are minimal side-effects from the skin pads (allergy, which can be reduced by using hypoallergic pads) or use of the current (can aggravate pain).

Interventional treatment of chronic pain

In the last decade or two, complex interventions for pain control have become common. Although interventions are more invasive than nerve blocks, many of them are not neurodestructive. These interventions can be neuromodulatory or neuroablative.

Neuromodulatory techniques

These techniques have the advantage of being reversible and therefore more appropriate for the treatment of non-malignant pain. They can be discontinued if they prove ineffective, without loss of any function. However, these procedures require expertise and highly technical infusion pumps and spinal cord stimulation systems. They also require more regular and frequent follow-up visits.

Neuromodulation (modulate pain signal prior to being received by brain) can be physical (electrical stimulation) or chemical (drugs).

Physical neuromodulation

Spinal cord stimulation (SCS). The aim of SCS is to relieve pain by applying sufficient electrical stimulation to cause paraesthesia covering or overlapping the area of pain without discomfort or motor effects. It does not affect acute pain sensation. An implanted pulse generator delivers a small amount of current to the spinal cord via a lead placed in the epidural space. This causes paraesthesia in the painful region by stimulating Aβ-fibres. Stimulation of Aβ-fibres and a descending inhibitory pathway 'closes the gate' in the dorsal horn of the spinal cord, which regulates transmission of pain to the brain. There is selective stimulation of dorsal column fibres without any effect on motor fibres.

SCS is used to treat chronic pain with a specific diagnosis, particularly of non-malignant origin. It is used only if less invasive treatment options have failed to relieve the pain. It remains popular despite the high cost of the hardware and its maintenance. SCS therapy has its own side-effects. Common and less serious complications are electrode migration, electrode breakage, system infection, system damage due to ingress of body fluids, system disconnection and post-dural puncture headache. Rare but serious complications are nerve root damage related to electrode placement, paraplegia from spinal haematoma and abscess.

The overall complication rate reported in the first 12 months following SCS system implantation is 43%, reducing to about 4% thereafter, so that most patients who benefit from SCS are able to continue using this therapy in the longer term. The complication rate is likely to be lower in a service with experienced implanting clinicians and a multidisciplinary team adhering to principles of best practice.

The common indications are refractory angina pain, failed back surgery syndrome, complex regional pain syndrome and ischaemic leg pain.

Peripheral nerve stimulation (PNS). PNS is indicated in the treatment of chronic neuropathic pain in the distribution of a peripheral nerve. Particular nerve involvement in a pain problem is confirmed by a predictive nerve block using local anaesthetic. Although the exact mechanism of action of PNS is not understood, it works on similar principles to that of SCS. A stimulating lead is implanted parallel to the nerve and stimulated as required using an implantable pulse generator. The common indication for this procedure is occipital neuralgia.

Chemical neuromodulation

Intrathecal drug delivery (ITDD). In this technique pain is reduced or eliminated by directly injecting certain medications into the intrathecal space that interfere with the transmission of pain. A subcutaneously implanted reservoir pump delivers the drugs through an implanted and tunnelled catheter into the intrathecal space. The commonly used medications are morphine, baclofen (for the treatment of spasticity in spinal cord injury patients) and local anaesthetics. As drug is delivered directly to the site of action, the required dose is a fraction of that required orally (1:300). This small dose reduces side-effects and improves patient compliance.

ITDD is highly technical and demanding, and has the potential for significant complications. The patient should have had multidisciplinary assessment and therapy prior to ITDD. In patients with appropriate indications ITDD is a very effective therapy.

The common indications are malignant pain, failed back surgery syndrome, chronic regional pain syndrome, and widespread body pain not responding to conventional and less invasive therapy.

Neuroablation

Neuroablation is intentional injury of a nerve by chemical, thermal or surgical means to relieve the pain. It is performed at various anatomical sites to relieve refractory cancer pain, but, because of its associated risks, it is used infrequently to treat non-malignant pain.

The main advantage is that it is a single intervention with no maintenance therapy. This may reduce the demand on healthcare systems in the long term. The risks and limitations include neurological deficit, neuritis, damage to non-targeted tissues and failure due to an overlapping nerve supply.

Pain relief is rarely permanent and averages only 3–6 months in a patient with stable disease. This is due to plasticity as cell bodies are usually spared.

Thermal neuroablation

Cryoanalgesia is an application of extreme cold to damage a nerve. This technique causes degeneration of the nerve axon without epineural or perineural damage.

A cryoprobe consists of an outer tube and smaller inner tube, which terminates in a fine nozzle, and works on a principle based on the expansion of compressed gas (carbon dioxide or nitrous oxide). Expansion of the gas causes a rapid decrease in temperature (to −70°C) at the probe tip, leading to formation of an ice ball around the exterior of the tip.

Cryoanalgesia is suitable for the painful conditions originating from small, well-localized lesions of peripheral nerves, e.g. neuroma.

The duration of pain relief after cryoanalgesia ranges from 2 weeks to 5 months.

Radiofrequency (RF) ablation is the destruction of nerves by application of heat. It involves inserting a small insulated electrode with an exposed tip within the tissue surrounding the target nerve. The tissue impedes the flow of current through the needle, causing the current to be dissipated as heat. This heat in the surrounding tissue destroys the nerve.

RF lesioning is indicated for the treatment of pain in a well-defined anatomical location with a clear understanding of neuroanatomy involved in nociception. A prognostic block using local anaesthetic is advised to assess the possible response to RF lesioning. Complications of this procedure include neurological deficits, deafferentation pain, neuritis and burn injury at breaks in the needle insulation.

Facet joint pain and trigeminal neuralgia are commonly treated using RF lesioning.

Chemical neuroablation

Neurolytic agents. Alcohol (50–95%) and phenol (5–10%) are used for neurolysis. Because of the permanent nature of nerve damage caused by these agents, they are used mostly in patients with malignant pain. The procedures in which neurolytic solutions are commonly used are coeliac plexus block (for chronic pancreatitis or cancer of the pancreas), trigeminal ganglion block (for trigeminal neuralgia), lumbar sympathetic block (for ischaemic pain due to peripheral vascular disease) and spinal analgesia (for denervation of a sensory area in patients with terminal cancer pain).

Surgical neuroablation

In general neurosurgical consultation is sought only after a patient's pain has proved refractory to all appropriate medical therapies.

Surgical ablative procedures are often considered the final rung on the pain treatment ladder, but in some instances they are procedures of choice. For example, phantom limb pain following spinal nerve root avulsion can be treated effectively by dorsal root entry zone (DREZ) lesioning. This involves neural tissue destruction as well as the potential loss of function that accompanies the destruction of nervous tissue. This is less of a concern in patients with a limited life span (malignant pain).

Miscellaneous

Vertebroplasty

This is a relatively new procedure, approved by the National Institute for Health and Clinical Excellence (NICE) for the treatment of back pain caused by vertebral collapse. The vertebral collapse can be the result of a metastatic deposit or osteoporosis. The procedure involves injection of cement within the collapsed vertebral body (*see* Figure 6.6) and is performed by a radiologist.

Other procedures for low back pain not yet commonly used are nucleoplasty and intradiscal electrothermal annuloplasty diathermy.

Figure 6.6 Vertebroplasty

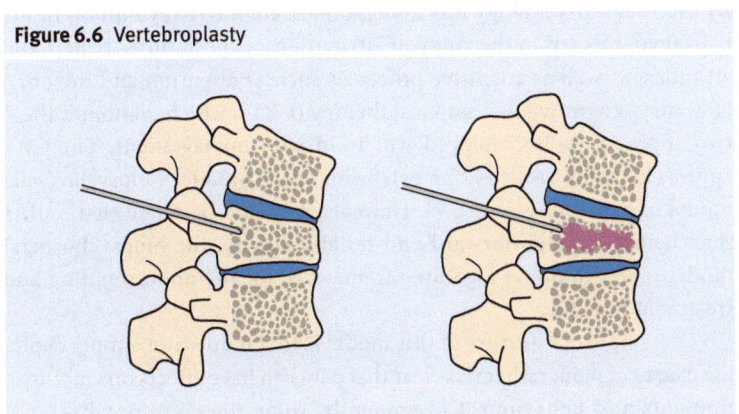

Rehabilitative and psychological approaches

Introduction

Psychological explanations of pain have a long history and over the years these have generated a number of treatment approaches. The earliest explanations were directed at understanding the occurrence of pain in the absence of physical pathology. These explanations focused on psychiatric problems or particular 'pain-prone' personality types as the causal agents. The treatments for this type of pain centred on the elimination of the particular psychopathology thought to be responsible. Pain therefore was thought to either be in the body or in the mind. Since the advent of the gate control theory (GCT) [6], this dualistic view of pain is seen as being outdated. The GCT postulated the existence of 'spinal gates' where descending cortical impulses could modulate or even block the transmission of afferent pain signals. Since the introduction of the GCT, an overwhelming body of evidence has accumulated that has demonstrated the extent to which the perception of pain is enmeshed in an individual's psychological and social situation.

At the time that the GCT was published, psychology was dominated by the behaviourist school. Behaviourism restricted itself to the study of observable phenomena and consequently subjective experiences, such as pain, were considered to be outside the realm of proper scientific analysis. However, 'pain behaviour' (guarding, grimacing, vocal expressions of pain, disability, etc.) is observable and therefore was thought to be open to proper scientific scrutiny. Fordyce [7] demonstrated in a series of experiments how pain behaviours can be shaped by environmental reinforcement, such as the concern of others and the avoidance of activity. By the 1980s, psychology was undergoing a 'cognitive revolution'. In the pain field, this led to the study of attributions, expectations, beliefs and attitudes, as well as cognitive processes such as attention and memory. Nowadays cognitive–behavioural therapy (CBT), which combines these two approaches, is employed widely in pain management. The CBT approach can be viewed as an extension of the broader biopsychosocial model of pain (*see* Figure 6.7). However it should be noted that, rather than being a straightforward and testable theory, the biopsychosocial model is seen more as a guiding framework for the understanding and treatment of pain.

One important feature of this model is that it does not simply depict the causes of pain; rather it is clear that pain can have effects on emotions, thoughts and behaviour. Consequently, some interventions have not

Figure 6.7 The biopsychosocial model

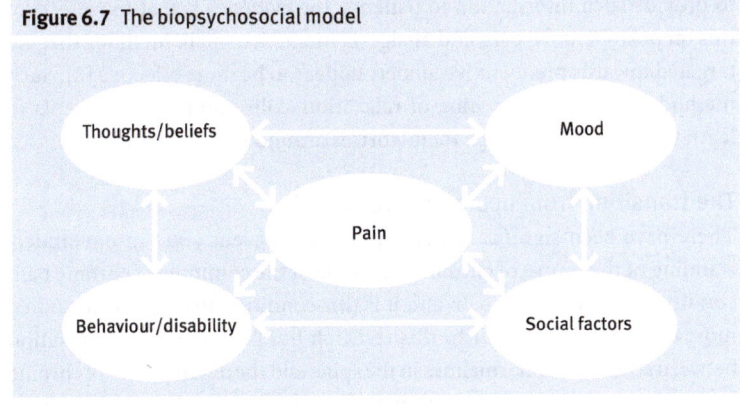

attempted to reduce pain but instead their aim has been to reduce the damage to an individual's quality of life that has resulted from enduring a life dominated by pain. Indeed, some authors are of the opinion that the struggle for pain control, when it is a chronic problem, is only ever likely to have limited success, but more importantly this struggle can actually be harmful to the enjoyment of life. Having said this, given that all the variables in the biopsychosocial model are thought to be causally interwoven, if an intervention results in improvements in an individual's mood and disability, it is also likely to lead to some improvement in their pain.

Acute/postoperative pain

Although most of this chapter is devoted to the management of chronic pain, it is worth mentioning briefly the psychological interventions that have been employed to help manage acute pain. There have been very many laboratory studies showing that psychological techniques are effective at moderating pain. However, the painful stimuli in these situations are generally mild in intensity and short-lived. While these studies are useful for helping to develop and test theory, their applicability to clinical situations, such as pain resulting from surgery or pain that is experienced during invasive procedures, is always open to question.

The simplest and most widely tested psychological intervention that has been conducted in hospital settings concerns the provision of information prior to surgery. The aim of such interventions has usually been to reduce anxiety about the procedure and to provide the patient with appropriate expectations about pain and the recovery process. While it is ethically crucial to provide such information to patients, the evidence is that the effects of this on postoperative pain and analgesia intake are small. Methods that are targeted towards preoperative anxiety appear to be more effective [8]. Such methods include the teaching of relaxation skills and helping patients to learn techniques to manage their worries around surgery better.

The transition from acute to chronic pain

There have been significant developments in recent years in our understanding of the causes of chronic pain. One of the commonest chronic pain conditions is lower back pain and it is this condition that has been studied most extensively. The spur to this research has been the poor association between structural abnormalities in the spine and the development of chronic low back pain. In contrast, a number of psychosocial predictors have been identified as being of crucial importance in making the transition from an acute episode of back pain and the development of a disabling, chronic problem. These psychosocial predictors have been termed the 'yellow flags' (*see* Figure 6.8). To a greater or lesser extent, these yellow flags have been implicated in other chronic pain conditions.

Attempts to prevent the development of chronic pain

There have been a number of public health campaigns conducted at various places around the world that have shown the beneficial effects of addressing some of these yellow flags with specific educational messages about back self-care [9]. Other researchers have focused their efforts on better understanding of

Figure 6.8 An overview of yellow flags

Belief that pain and activity are harmful

Sickness behaviours (like extended rest)

Low or negative moods, social withdrawal

Treatment that does not fit best practice

Problems with claims and compensation

History of back pain, time off, other claims

Problems at work, poor job satisfaction

Heavy work, unsociable hours

Overprotective family or lack of support

Reproduced with permission from: The Accident Compensation Corporation and the New Zealand Guidelines Group. New Zealand Acute Low Back Pain Guide: Incorporating the Guide to Assessing Psychosocial Yellow Flags in Acute Back Pain. Wellington, New Zealand: The Accident Compensation Corporation and the New Zealand Guidelines Group, 2003. (Available online at http://www.nzgg.org.nz/guidelines/0072/albp_guide_col.pdf). Last accessed 28 January 2008.

some of the maladaptive pain beliefs and their associated fears. Johan Vlaeyen and Steven Linton [10] have developed a cognitive–behavioural model of the fear of pain and how such fears might result in further pain and disability (*see* Figure 6.9). This model, which sees pain-related fear as having significant similarities to phobic states, appears to hold up well when its components are investigated in detail [11]. A series of case studies have been published by the authors where these fears have been reduced successfully using education and carefully planned, graded exposure to feared movements.

Psychological methods of controlling pain

A recent Cochrane library review by Raymond Ostello and his colleagues [12] divided these psychological methods into four categories: operant techniques, respondent techniques, cognitive techniques and a final category containing different combinations of these three types.

Operant techniques are those pioneered by Fordyce and include positive reinforcement of healthy behaviours alongside a withdrawal of attention towards pain behaviours. Ostello and colleagues managed to locate only three randomized controlled trials of sufficient quality to include in their review. They concluded that these trials either showed little difference in pain and functioning compared with controls, or that the evidence was insufficient to settle the question.

Figure 6.9 Cognitive–behavioural model of pain-related fear

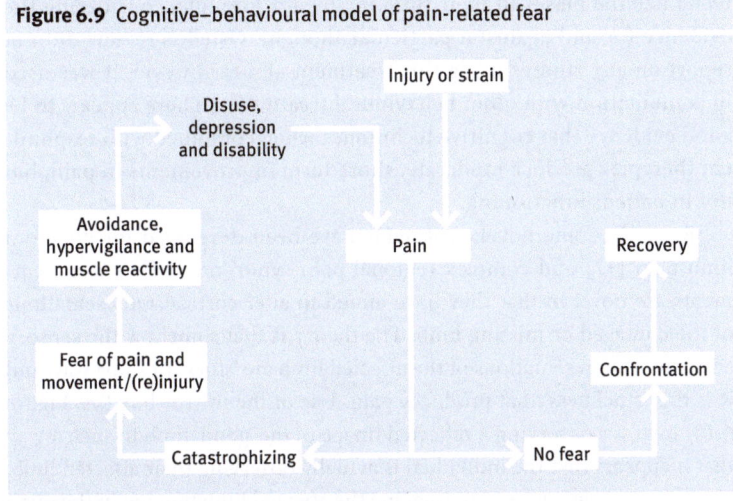

Reproduced with permission from: Vlaeyen JWS, Kole-Snidjers AMJ, Boeren RGB, van Eek H. Fear of movement/(re)injury in chronic low back pain patients: an experimental investigation. Pain 1995; 62:363–72.

Respondent techniques aim to modify the physiological response directly. Included in this class of techniques are progressive muscular relaxation, applied relaxation and electromyography biofeedback. These techniques aim to reduce muscular tension, which is thought to aggravate pain, and replace it with an incompatible relaxed state. The relaxation treatments involve encouraging the patient to focus systematically on various muscle groups and to become more aware of what a relaxed muscular state feels like, the theory being that it becomes easier following training to return the body to this state. Ostello's systematic review concluded that there was moderate evidence that relaxation has a large positive effect on pain and functioning, at least in the short term.

Electromyography biofeedback works by providing information to the individual on the extent of muscular tension in their body. This feedback is usually in an audible (for example, a rising or falling tone) or visual (for example, a flashing light) form, and is of a degree of precision that is not usually available to conscious awareness. With training the individual is thought to achieve a greater degree of voluntary control over muscular tension than they had before training. Unfortunately, Ostello and his colleagues concluded that there is insufficient evidence that this technique relieves pain or improves functioning. Cognitive techniques aim to modify maladaptive cognitions, either indirectly, using techniques such as imagery or distraction, or by teaching the individual to recognize the biases in their thinking by, for example, considering the evidence for and against a particular thought. Ostello's review did not report on any studies using this treatment alone; however, it was used in combination with other behavioural treatments. There appears to be good evidence that cognitive techniques when combined with respondent therapies produce moderate, short-term improvements in pain, but not in patient functioning.

Recently, some novel treatments have been developed for phantom limb pain [13] and complex regional pain syndrome [14]. These treatments are novel in that they have aimed to alter cortical representations of the damaged or missing limb. The theory is that somehow the sensory and motor representations of the affected limb are 'stuck' in some way, and it is this 'stuckness' that produces pain. Use of the mirror box (see Figure 6.10) involves observing a reflected image of the 'good' limb in such a way that it appears that the individual is actually observing their affected limb. They are then encouraged to imagine the affected limb moving in the same way as the image is. It is thought that this procedure helps to 'reassure' the sensory and motor cortex that 'all is well' with the affected limb. Although

Figure 6.10 A mirror box

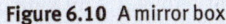

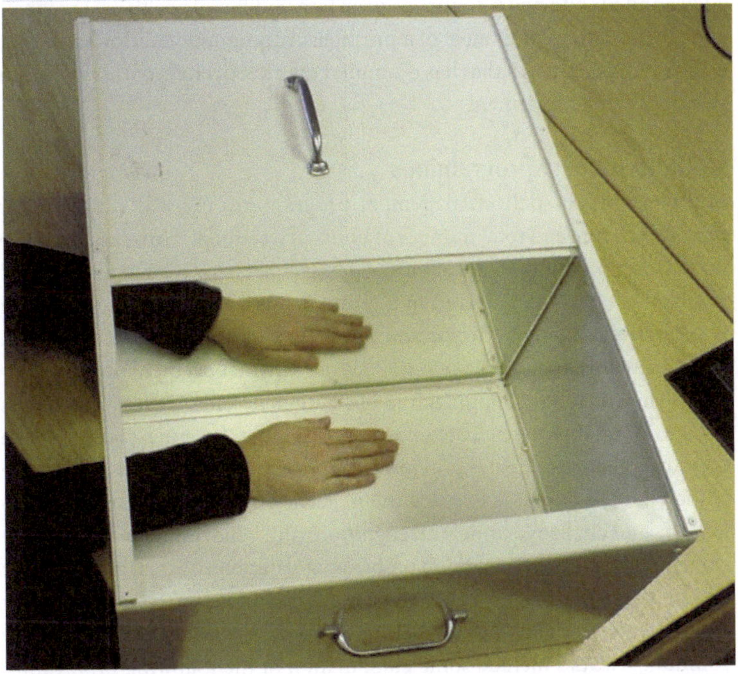

interesting from a theoretical perspective, it is perhaps a little early to be confident about the effectiveness of this approach.

Rehabilitative approaches

These can be separated into uni-disciplinary interventions, usually focusing on one aspect of the condition (for example, the physical restrictions that accompany pain), or more intensive, multidisciplinary programmes.

Exercise is the single most common rehabilitative approach for chronic musculoskeletal pain, ideally guided by a physiotherapist. The evidence in non-specific low back pain is that this is helpful in comparison to usual care, although a gentle and general exercise programme is preferable to specific back exercises [15]. There has been some concern that individuals with high levels of fear-avoidance beliefs will fail to improve with this approach.

Activity pacing focuses on increasing the level of daily activity and replacing activity contingent on pain with activity contingent on a planned quota. Other aspects of pacing include setting low-activity baselines at the beginning, breaking activities into manageable parts, increasing the amount of activity gradually and alternating between different activities. This kind of advice and monitoring is routinely given by a number of health professionals and is frequently a component of more intensive programmes. However, there is little published work that has examined the effectiveness of this approach as a stand-alone treatment.

Multidisciplinary programmes

Multidisciplinary pain management programmes (PMPs) vary in their content, staffing and total number of hours of treatment. However, there are some commonalities. PMPs are usually based on cognitive and behavioural principles. They are delivered in a group format, and active participation is strongly encouraged. Common components of PMPs include education about pain physiology, pain psychology and self-management of pain problems. The educational approach is not a didactic one; rather participants are encouraged to participate and reflect on how these messages apply to their own histories. Help is provided to set functional goals and patients are guided in their attempts to reach them. Participants in PMPs are helped to identify and challenge unhelpful cognitions and behavioural habits that are contributing to their pain, mood problems and disability. Stress management and lifestyle advice is provided and a graded exercise programme of light-to-moderate intensity is usually an integral part. Staffing varies but most commonly would include some combination of the following professions: clinical psychology, physiotherapy, medicine (most commonly an anaesthetist, rheumatologist or rehabilitation consultant), nursing, occupational therapy and pharmacy, although some programmes will include other professions not listed here.

These programmes are usually evaluated as a whole package and comparisons made with waiting list controls or care as usual [16]. While these evaluations provide good evidence that these kinds of treatments reduce pain, improve mood and lessen disability, there is work still to be done examining the effects of matching treatment programmes to specific patient characteristics [17].

Many PMPs have employed the CBT model to good effect in helping chronic pain sufferers regain some control over their lives, although recent theorists have argued that it is the struggle to control pain, as well as the struggle to control thoughts, emotions and behaviour, that is often behind much of the harm caused by having pain. Acceptance and commitment therapy (ACT) shifts the focus of treatment from one of control to one where individuals are encouraged to develop a willingness to experience unpleasant private experiences without having to do anything about them. One of the advantages of this 'acceptance' is that it is thought to allow the individual to regain a sense of self that is not completely entangled with their identity as a pain sufferer and to enable the pursuit of valued goals. A review of studies applying this approach to the pain field [18] suggests that ACT has the potential to be a valuable addition to current psychological treatment approaches.

References

1. Benzon HT. Epidural steroids injection for low back pain and lumbosacral radiculopathy. Pain 1986; 24:277–95.
2. Wallace M, Staats P. Pain Medicine and Management: Just the Facts. Maidenhead: McGraw-Hill Professional, 2004.
3. Prithvi Raj P (ed.). Practical Management of Pain, 3rd edn. St Louis, MO: Mosby, 2000.
4. Kanner R (ed.). Pain Management Secrets, 2nd edn. Philadelphia: Hanley & Belfus, 2003.
5. National Institute for Health and Clinical Excellence. Percutaneous vertebroplasty, IP Guidance Number IPG12. London: NICE, September 2003 (available from http://www.nice.org.uk/nicemedia/pdf/ip/IPG012guidance.pdf). Last accessed 8 January 2008.
6. Melzack R, Wall PD. Pain mechanisms: a new theory. Science 1965; 150:171–9.
7. Fordyce WE. A behavioural perspective on chronic pain. Br J Clin Psychol 1982; 21:313–20.
8. Johnston M, Vogele C. What benefits can psychological preparation for surgery achieve? Ann Behav Med 1993; 15:245–56.
9. Buchbinder R, Jolley D, Wyatt M. Population based interventions to change back beliefs and disability: a three part evaluation. BMJ 2001; 322:1516–20.
10. Vlaeyen JWS, Linton SJ. Fear-avoidance and its consequences in chronic musculoskeletal pain: a state of the art. Pain 2000; 85:317–32.
11. Leeuw M, Goossens MEJB, Linton SJ, et al. The fear-avoidance model of musculoskeletal pain: current state of scientific evidence. J Behav Med 2007; 30:77–94.
12. Ostelo RWJG, van Tulder MW, Vlaeyen JWS, et al. Behavioural treatment for chronic low back pain. Cochrane Database of Systematic Reviews 2000 (2); CD002014.
13. Ramachandran VS, Blakeslee S. Phantoms in the Brain: Probing the Mysteries of the Human Mind. New York: William Morrow, 1998.
14. Moseley L. Graded motor imagery for pathologic pain: a randomized controlled trial. Neurology 2006; 67:2129–34.
15. Hayden JA, van Tulder MW, Malmivaara A, et al. Exercise therapy for treatment of non-specific low back pain. Cochrane Database of Systematic Reviews 2000 (3); CD000335.
16. Morley S, Eccleston C, Williams A. Systematic review and meta-analysis of randomized controlled trials of cognitive behaviour therapy and behaviour therapy for chronic pain in adults, excluding headache. Pain 2000; 80:1–13.
17. Vlaeyen JWS, Morley S. Cognitive-behavioural treatments for chronic pain: what works for whom? Clin J Pain 2005; 21(1):1–8.
18. McCracken LM, Vowles KE. Acceptance of chronic pain. Curr Pain Headache Rep 2006; 10:90–4.

Index